O E L

OXFORD ENDOCRINOLOGY LIBRARY

Testosterone
Deficiency in Men

D1560302

O E L

OXFORD ENDOCRINOLOGY LIBRARY

Testosterone Deficiency in Men

Edited by

T. Hugh Jones

Consultant Physician and Endocrinologist,
Honorary Professor of Andrology,
Barnsley Hospital and the University of Sheffield, UK

OXFORD
UNIVERSITY PRESS

OXFORD
UNIVERSITY PRESS

Great Clarendon Street, Oxford OX2 6DP

Oxford University Press is a department of the University of Oxford.
It furthers the University's objective of excellence in research, scholarship,
and education by publishing worldwide in

Oxford New York

Auckland Cape Town Dar es Salaam Hong Kong Karachi
Kuala Lumpur Madrid Melbourne Mexico City Nairobi
New Delhi Shanghai Taipei Toronto

With offices in

Argentina Austria Brazil Chile Czech Republic France Greece
Guatemala Hungary Italy Japan Poland Portugal Singapore
South Korea Switzerland Thailand Turkey Ukraine Vietnam

Oxford is a registered trade mark of Oxford University Press
in the UK and in certain other countries

Published in the United States
by Oxford University Press Inc., New York

British Library Cataloguing in Publication Data
Data available

Library of Congress Cataloging in Publication Data
Data available

Typeset by Newgen Imaging Systems (P) Ltd., Chennai, India
Printed in Italy
on acid-free paper by
L.E.G.O. S.p.A – Lavis TN

ISBN 978-0-19-954513-1

10 9 8 7 6 5 4 3 2 1

Whilst every effort has been made to ensure that the contents of this book are as
complete, accurate and-up-to-date as possible at the date of writing. Oxford
University Press is not able to give any guarantee or assurance that such is the case.
Readers are urged to take appropriately qualified medical advice in all cases. The
information in this book is intended to be useful to the general reader, but should
not be used as a means of self-diagnosis or for the prescription of medication.

Contents

Foreword

Since its isolation and chemical synthesis in the 1930's testosterone has always been a hormone surrounded by uncertainty and controversy.

Apart from its well-known beneficial actions on libido, sexual performance, mood, muscle strength, and bone in patients with primary and secondary hypogonadism, testosterone dreams about rejuvenation, its uses as an aphrodisiac and in doping have been extensively discussed in the lay press for more than sixty years.

It is for this reason that Professor Hugh Jones is to be applauded for his initiative in editing a book directed at primary, as well as secondary care physicians which aims to increase knowledge and awareness of the optimal diagnosis and treatment of hypogonadism.

In this book the 'classical' knowledge about signs, symptoms and diagnostic evaluation of primary and secondary hypogonadism is well-presented together with the newest insights in the application of the different testosterone formulations which are presently available.

Testosterone levels fall after the age of 40 by 1 to 2% per year. In recent years a lively debate has been carried out about androgen deficiency in ageing males and the definition of 'late-onset hypogonadism'. In this book a number of contributors present the guidelines for this diagnosis and its treatment in a balanced manner, putting the role of the metabolic syndrome, type 2 diabetes mellitus and other co-morbidities in perspective as well. Also the beneficial actions of testosterone therapy in angina pectoris and heart failure are well presented.

Testosterone is the hormone which elicits more imagination, dreams, and uncertainty than any other hormone. This book provides excellent state-of-the-art guidance to all health care professionals on how to make an optimal diagnosis of hypogonadism, as well as how to treat patients.

Steven W.J. Lamberts
Professor of Medicine
Erasmus Medical Center
Rotterdam
The Netherlands

Preface

'Medicine is an art based on science.' Sir William Osler, 1892.

Male hypogonadism, the clinical syndrome of testosterone deficiency is an under-recognized and under-diagnosed medical condition. The reasons for this include the non-specificity of symptoms, difficulties in the interpretation of the biochemical tests, a lack of clinical awareness and concerns over prostate safety. There is little doubt however, that hypogonadism is an important condition for the medical practitioner to diagnose. Many men with symptoms of testosterone deficiency will first present to the primary care physician but will also come into the realms of specific secondary care health professionals which include diabetologists, endocrinologists, sexual medicine, cardiologists, medicine for the elderly physicians, urologists, genito-urinary physicians, orthopaedic surgeons, psychiatrists and psychologists.

This book, as part of the *Oxford Endocrinology Library*, provides not only a reference to the classical knowledge of hypogonadism but also builds on this by providing up-to-date current opinion based on a wealth of recent publications in medical literature. Importantly, international guidelines for the diagnosis and management of hypogonadism have been published. There are however grey areas where the diagnosis may be unclear and this is where the art of the physician comes into play. One of the major recent advances is the availability of pharmaceutical preparations, which allow testosterone to be replaced to normal physiological levels.

Hypogonadism is associated with a reduced quality of life and well-being, and can result in loss of livelihood and difficulties between partners, leading to separation. Recent evidence has found that testosterone deficiency is also an independent risk factor for the future development of the metabolic syndrome and type 2 diabetes. An increased prevalence of low testosterone levels in men has been associated with several chronic medical disorders, which for example include diabetes, cardiovascular disease, chronic obstructive pulmonary disease, osteoporosis, frailty, depression, erectile dysfunction and HIV infection. Chapters on these specific disease areas discuss the current state of knowledge. It is important to note that in the majority of these conditions the role of testosterone replacement therapy needs to be determined by the commission of larger and longer-term clinical trials. However, the benefits of testosterone treatment for hypogonadal men are recognized with regard to improvements in sexual function, body composition and bone mineral density.

PREFACE

I wish to thank the contributors to this book who are all key opinion leaders and active researchers in the field. It is my hope that this book will be informative and enlighten all members of the medical profession and other interested health professionals. This would then lead to an increase in clinical awareness, diagnosis and treatment of hypogonadism, which could in turn result in significant and in some cases dramatic improvement in their patients' quality of life and wellbeing.

Hugh Jones,
April 2008

Contributors

Bradley D. Anawalt,
Associate Chief of Medicine, VA Puget Sound Healthcare System, Seattle and Professor of Medicine, University of Washington, USA

Stefan Arver,
Director and Associate Professor, Centre for Andrology and Sexual Medicine Department of Endocrinology, Metabolism and Diabetes Karolinska University Hospital and Karolinska Institute, Stockholm, Sweden

Hermann Behre,
Director, Center of Reproductive Medicine and Andrology, University Hospital Halle, Halle, Germany

Shalender Bhasin,
Professor of Medicine and Chief of Endocrinology, Diabetes and Nutrition, Boston University School of Medicine, Section of Endocrinology, Diabetes and Nutrition, Boston Medical Center, Boston, USA

Pierre-Marc Bouloux,
Professor of Endocrinology, Centre for Neuroendocrinology, Royal Free and University College Medical School, Hampstead, London, UK

Ahmed El-Sakka,
Department of Urology, Suez Canal University, School of Medicine, Ismailia, Egypt and Al-Noor Specialist Hospital, Makkah, Saudi Arabia

Arif Hambda,
Specialist Registrar Centre for Neuroendocrinology, Royal Free and University College Medical School, Hampstead, London, UK

Trudy Hannington,
Sexual Therapist, Leger Clinic, St. Vincent Medical Centre, Doncaster, UK

T. Hugh Jones,
Consultant Physician and Endocrinologist and Honorary Professor of Andrology, Robert Hague Centre for Diabetes and Endocrinology, Barnsley Hospital NHS Foundation Trust, Barnsley, and Academic Unit of Diabetes, Endocrinology and Metabolism, The Medical School, University of Sheffield, Sheffield, UK

Mikael Lehtihet,
Centre for Andrology and Sexual Medicine Department of Endocrinology, Metabolism and Diabetes Karolinska University Hospital and Karolinska Institute, Stockholm, Sweden

Farid Saad,
Professor and Head of Global
Scientific Affairs, Bayer Schering
Pharma, Scientific Affairs Men's
Healthcare, Berlin, Germany,
and Gulf Medical University
School of Medicine, Ajman,
United Arab Emirates.

Doug Savage,
General Practitioner,
Leger Clinic, St. Vincent
Medical Centre,
Doncaster, UK

Aksam Yassin,
Consultant Urologist and
Professor of Urology and
Human Sexuality, Segeburger
Kliniken, Norderstedt-Hamburg,
Germany and Gulf Medical
University School of medicine,
Ajman, United Arab Emirates.

Michael Zitzmann,
Clinical Director, Institute of
Reproductive Medicine,
Universitaksklinikum Munster,
Munster, Germany

Symbols and abbreviations

ARE	androgen response element
BLSA	Baltimore Longitudinal Study of Aging
cAMP	cyclic adenosine monophosphate
CHD	coronary heart disease
eNOS	endothelial nitric oxide synthase
EAU	European Association of Urology
ED	erectile dysfunction
eNOS	endothelial nitric oxide synthase
FSH	follicle-stimulating hormone
GnRH	gonadotrophin-releasing hormone
hCG	human chorionic gonadotrophin
HDL	high-density lipoprotein
hMG	human menopause gonadatrophin
HOMA-IR	homeostatic model assessment of insulin resistance
HRT	hormone replacement therapy
HUVEC	human umbilical vein endothelial cells
ICSI	intracytoplasmic sperm injection
IDF	International Diabetes Federation
IHH	Isolated Hypogonadotrophic Hypogonadism
IIEF	International Index of Erectile Function
IPPS	International Prostate Symptom Score
ISA	International Society of Andrology
ISSAM	International Society for the Study of the Aging Male
LBM	lean body mass
LDL	low density lipoprotein
LH	luteinizing hormone
MMAS	Massachusetts Male Aging Study
MRFIT	Multiple Risk Factor Intervention Trial
NANC	non-adrenergic-noncholinergic neurons
NCEP III	National Cholesterol Education Program Expert Panel III

NHANES III	National Health and Nutrition Survey III
nNOS	neural nitric oxide synthase
NO	nitric oxide
PAI-1	plasminogen-activator inhibitor type 1
PDE-5	phosphodiesterase type 5
PSA	prostate-specific antigen
SARM	selective androgen receptor modulators
SHBG	sex hormone-binding globulin
tPA	tissue plasminogen activator
TNF	tumour necrosis factor
TU	testosterone undecanoate
UQCRB	ubiquinol cytochrome c reductase-binding protein
VCAM-1	vascular adhesion molecule type 1
VGCCs	voltage-gated calcium channels
WHO	World Health Organization

Chapter 1

Testosterone deficiency: an overview

T. Hugh Jones

> **Key points**
>
> - Hypogonadism is an underdiagnosed condition.
> - There needs to be an increased clinical awareness among medical and health professionals in general.
> - Men with hypogonadism may present to a wide range of medical specialities.
> - Low testosterone levels are associated with increased morbidity and mortality.
> - Advances in testosterone delivery enable replacement to physiological levels.

1.1 Introduction

Over recent years, testosterone has been perceived by a large proportion of clinicians as predominantly a sex hormone. However, recent research has demonstrated that testosterone has important biological effects, in particular, on metabolism, bone, and muscle integrity, the cardiovascular system, and the brain. There is now good evidence that testosterone deficiency causes: (1) reduced insulin sensitivity and impaired carbohydrate metabolism; (2) increased bone turnover; (3) muscle weakness; (4) impaired cognitive function; (5) and reduced motivational drive, as well as fatigue and lethargy.

Male hypogonadism is a recognized medical condition that remains underdiagnosed by clinicians. Klinefelter's Syndrome is the commonest classical cause of hypogonadism (1 in 660 male births); however a Danish registry study has demonstrated that only 1 in 4 cases is diagnosed. A similar experience was reported in the UK from the North Thames Congenital Malformation Register where only 1 in 4 cases were detected postnatally. In 2000 it was estimated in the USA that only 1 in 20 subjects with hypogonadism was diagnosed and treated. This is likely to be reflected in other countries in the Western world.

There are several reasons why hypogonadism is underdiagnosed: (1) patients may not present to their health professional because they may feel embarrassed and reserved about their symptoms because of their sexual nature, or they just believe that they are a consequence of getting older; (2) patients may present to their doctor with non-specific symptoms, such as tiredness, lack of motivation, anxiety, or depression, which may have occurred directly as a result of marital difficulties due to sexual problems; (3) the symptoms of hypogonadism are non-specific and can be frequently manifestations of other medical conditions; (4) there is no definitive biochemical test for hypogonadism and unless the testosterone level is significantly below normal it can be difficult to interpret; and (5) there is a general lack of clinical awareness of the condition.

Hypogonadism can lead to a significant reduction in quality of life, the loss of livelihood, and disharmony between partners. It may also present with lethargy and fatigue to a similar degree as primary hypothyroidism. This symptom can be profound. Measurement of testosterone is not routinely performed in the work-up of a patient presenting with tiredness, but thyroid function is universally assessed. It is suggested that if the initial screen for the causes of tiredness is negative, and on systematic enquiry there is at least one other symptom consistent with hypogonadism, a testosterone level should be requested. It is acknowledged that if the testosterone level is low it could be related to the presence of another illness but would warrant appropriate investigation.

The primary care physician is usually the first contact with the medical profession and there does need to be an increased clinical awareness of the condition and its associations. Equally, men with hypogonadism may present to: orthopaedic surgeons with osteoporosis or fractures; urologists, sexual medicine doctors, or diabetologists with erectile dysfunction; psychologists or psychiatrists with depression; cardiologists and endocrinologists with metabolic syndrome. In addition, the couple may present to the infertility clinic or indeed the female partner may present alone.

1.2 **Making a diagnosis of hypogonadism**

This is not straightforward and is discussed in detail in Chapter 3. The problems arise because the symptoms are non-specific and there is no biochemical test with a clear cut-off between normal and abnormal. Assessment of levels of total testosterone remains the mainstay of the initial investigation; however, in borderline cases it can be helpful to assess free or bioavailable testosterone. Normal ranges of testosterone are usually based on a cohort of young healthy men. Age-specific ranges are not quoted, however; the value of these is unclear. It is apparent, however, that some men who have testosterone levels in the lower part of the normal range (8–12 nmol/l) do have hypogonadal symptoms, which respond to testosterone substitution. International guidelines are now in place, which act as an aid to making the diagnosis. In some patients where there is a high clinical suspicion and borderline testosterone values a clinical trial of testosterone replacement therapy may be warranted.

1.3 Androgenization

The state of androgenization in an individual will be a product of the delivery of testosterone to the tissues, its local metabolism and breakdown, and the cellular sensitivity to the hormone. The key components that affect this are the circulating testosterone level, the proportion of biologically active hormone, the sensitivity of the androgen receptor, the tissue levels of co-activators for the receptor; also the expression and activity of specific enzymes that metabolize testosterone and the local importance of non-genomic actions. New evidence has found that androgen receptor sensitivity can differ within populations. Furthermore, in individuals with the more insensitive receptor their testosterone levels are higher to compensate for this. This underlines the potential importance of pharmacogenetics in the management of hypogonadism.

1.4 Advances in testosterone replacement therapy

A major advance in testosterone replacement therapy was the development of formulations that allow testosterone to be replaced to physiological levels. Older treatments (e.g. testosterone ester intramuscular injections and implants) initially produced supraphysiological levels that were sometimes very high, declining gradually and then falling to the subphysiological range before the next treatment. These wide fluctuations in some individuals led to significant changes in symptoms especially when levels fell below the normal range. In particular, the gel, buccal, and long-acting intramuscular preparations, some of which allowed dose adjustments, achieved replacement to physiological levels. However, none of the preparations mimic exactly the circadian rhythm of testosterone.

1.5 Prostate safety

Many of the side-effects of testosterone listed in drug data sheets and formularies are based on the older generation of testosterone preparations. The more modern formulations are better tolerated and have fewer side-effects. The main concern of many doctors has been that of prostate carcinoma. There are no long-term controlled trials of testosterone therapy that can provide a definitive assessment of risk. However, a large number of smaller trials and longer-term population studies do not support the historical premise that testosterone replacement therapy increases the risk of prostate carcinoma. Indeed there is accumulating evidence, that low testosterone levels are associated with a greater risk of the occurrence of more aggressive prostate cancers. Provided the presence of prostate carcinoma is excluded before starting testosterone replacement therapy and patients are carefully monitored, as defined by guidelines, then with the available evidence concern should be allayed. It is, however, important that the patient is fully educated regarding this issue and the decision to treat is agreed by both the patient and the doctor.

1.6 **Morbidity and mortality**

In men with Klinefelter's Syndrome there is an increased risk of (1) being admitted to hospital and (2) dying from lung cancer, diabetes, circulatory, cerebrovascular and respiratory disease, and vascular insufficiency of the intestine. Klinefelter's Syndrome is also associated with a greater prevalence of osteoporosis, thromboembolic disease, glucose intolerance and diabetes, mediastinal tumours, mitral valve prolapse, and autoimmune rheumatological disorders, in particular, systemic lupus erythematosus. These findings alone should be enough to galvanize the clinician's mind to being alert to the condition. Furthermore, the association of major disease conditions, (which may have implications for morbidity and mortality) with a state of testosterone deficiency clearly raises the question, 'Why?'

The association of low testosterone levels with increased mortality has been confirmed in four population studies reported in 2006 and 2007. First, a study of American veterans in Seattle followed for up to 8 years after hospital admission found that a low testosterone level led to an increased risk of death from all-cause mortality. There was also an increased risk of death related to cardiovascular disease, diabetes, and respiratory conditions. This finding was supported by a study of an older population of community dwelling men, (the Rancho Bernado study), who also had an increase in all-cause mortality correlated with lower testosterone levels over a 20-year follow-up period (mean 11.8 years). The low testosterone group as a whole had a 33% greater chance of dying over an 18-year period than a man with higher testosterone levels. The low testosterone levels predicted an increased risk of cardiovascular and respiratory disease mortality. A study of 11,606 men from Norfolk, UK, also found that testosterone levels were inversely related to all-cause mortality, cardiovascular disease and cancer. The Massachusetts Male Aging Study, which included younger men (40–70 years), showed a weak association of low testosterone with a risk of premature death.

The Caerphilly study found that men who shaved less often than daily have a 52% higher risk of cardiovascular mortality over 20 years than men who shaved daily after adjustment for age. This study also found a specific association of both a high cortisol to testosterone ratio, as well as a weak association of testosterone, with incident ischaemic heart disease.

1.7 Co-morbidities

There is accumulating evidence that testosterone deficiency is associated with a number of common medical conditions that include cardiovascular, cerebrovascular, respiratory and renal disease, the metabolic syndrome and diabetes, osteoporosis, Alzheimer's disease, autoimmune disease, and HIV infection. It is unclear whether or not the low testosterone levels occur in these conditions, either: (1) as a consequence of suppression of the hypothalamic–pituitary–testicular axis, which is as a result of the associated inflammatory response caused by the disease process; (2) as a pre-existing state of testosterone deficiency; or (3) as a combination of these factors. Longitudinal population studies have clearly demonstrated that a low testosterone level is an independent risk factor for the later development of metabolic syndrome and type 2 diabetes. Klinefelter's Syndrome also predisposes to the conditions above and supports the premise that pre-existing testosterone deficiency is a risk factor for these disorders. Metabolic syndrome and diabetes are associated with cardiovascular risk and by extrapolation suggest that low testosterone state is in itself a cardiovascular risk factor. The likelihood is that testosterone deficiency is involved as a combination of cause and consequence.

1.8 Benefits on the immune system

There have been a number of case reports over the last 50 years or so in which testosterone therapy has been reported to improve inflammatory clinical conditions, e.g. rheumatoid arthritis and systemic lupus erythematosus. There is now recent evidence that demonstrates that testosterone replacement therapy suppresses the circulating levels of pro-inflammatory cytokines and promotes the production of anti-inflammatory cytokines in men with coronary heart disease and diabetes. An important study found that testosterone directly modulates the production of inflammatory cytokines from antigen-presenting cells. These exciting findings set a platform for further research to study the mechanisms and importance of normal circulating testosterone levels on the immune system.

1.9 **Potential benefits of testosterone replacement**

1.9.1 **Erectile dysfunction**

The role of testosterone in normal erectile function is becoming increasingly clear. Testosterone is critical in the maintenance of normal penile architecture and vascular flow. This is supported clinically by the finding that restoration of testosterone levels can convert just over half of sildenafil failures into sildenafil responders.

1.9.2 **Cardiovascular disease**

As long ago as 1939–46 (even reported in *TIME* magazine in 1942), there were several reports that testosterone treatment improved the symptoms of angina and intermittent claudication. The main medical pioneers of this treatment were Drs Maurice Aaron Lesser and Leslie Hamm from the USA. These important findings appeared to have been lost in the mists of medical history but recent studies have confirmed these discoveries. There is convincing evidence to support the action of testosterone as an arterial vasodilator.

The higher mortality risk in men compared with women has not been satisfactorily accounted for. Several studies have found that there is a high prevalence of low testosterone levels in cardiovascular disease. It is not clear if this is a contributory factor to atherogenesis or a consequence of the disease. It is likely, however, that it is a combination of these factors. Testosterone deficiency is associated with several cardiovascular risk factors, which include visceral obesity, insulin resistance, dyslipidaemia, hypertension, and prothrombotic and proatherogenic cytokine profiles. It is important to recognize that the pathogenesis of cardiovascular disease is multifactorial and that individual risk factors will have different weighting of importance between individuals.

Whether or not testosterone substitution improves overall cardiovascular risk remains to be shown; however, short-term studies have been favourable. Furthermore, studies using animal models have demonstrated that testosterone deficiency promotes atherogenesis and replacement protects against its development and also can reverse some changes.

In women, hormone replacement therapy (HRT) in the Women's Health Initiative Study found that there was an increase in thromboembolic events in the older woman. This may raise some concern with regard to testosterone. Testosterone administration has, however, not been shown to have any adverse effects on clotting and, conversely, in some studies has shown benefit. In addition, the hormones given to women in HRT preparations are not naturally occurring substances.

1.9.3 **Diabetes mellitus**

There is a high prevalence of hypogonadism in men with type 2 diabetes that is underdiagnosed. Appropriate treatment of the hypogonadism leads to resolution of hypogonadal symptoms and, importantly, improvement in quality of life. In addition, recent albeit short-term pilot studies have found that testosterone substitution improves insulin resistance, glycaemic control, waist circumference, and hypercholesterolaemia. As with cardiovascular disease larger and longer-term studies are needed to fully evaluate any benefits or risks.

1.10 **Age**

Circulating testosterone levels fall with age; however, the rate of decline varies between individuals. In many men testosterone levels do not fall into the hypogonadal range until after their 7th decade. In the presence of a diagnosis of hypogonadism an underlying cause should be sought. If no cause is found then the diagnosis of late-onset hypogonadism can be made according to international guidelines. Informed discussion with the patient should occur and a decision between patient and doctor considered regarding treatment.

There are several potential benefits of testosterone substitution in men with late-onset hypogonadism, which include prevention and treatment of osteoporosis, improvement in muscle strength and reduction in frailty. The health economic cost of frailty and immobility due to osteoporosis is high and will increase with an ever-ageing population. As described above there are also promising indications that testosterone replacement has benefits in cardiovascular disease. Although it is too early to say, it is however, conceivable that normalization of testosterone could have a significant effect on cerebral function.

1.11 **Conclusions**

Testosterone is a naturally occurring hormone, which if replaced to physiological levels can have major clinical effects on a range of factors that improve well-being and quality of life as well as potentially enhancing life expectancy. It must be stated that nowadays any clinical benefits and safety issues have to be proven in long-term clinical trials. There is now enough evidence from epidemiological and short-term studies to support the commissioning of long-term trials. However, a greater clinical confidence has arisen by the development of new testosterone formulations, which allow fairly accurate restoration of normal physiology. It is important to consider and discuss the benefits versus risks in any individual patient. If the decision to treat is carefully made, contraindications excluded, and treatment monitored, then the current evidence suggests that testosterone replacement therapy is safe and may well be cost-effective.

Key references

Araujo AB, Kupelian V, Page ST et al. (2007). Sex steroids and all-cause mortality and cause-specific mortality in men. *Arch Int Med* **167**: 1252–60.

Bojesen A, Juul S, Birkebæk NH, Gravholt CH. (2006). Morbidity in Klinefelter syndrome: a Danish register study based on hospital discharge diagnoses. *J Clin Endocrinol Metab* **91**: 1254–60.

Keating NL, O'Malley J, Smith MR. (2006). Diabetes and cardiovascular disease during androgen deprivation therapy for prostate cancer. *J Clin Oncol* **24**: 4448–56.

Khaw K, Dowsett M, Folkerd E, et al. (2007). Endogenous testosterone and mortality due to all causes, cardiovascular disease, and cancer in men. European prospective investigation into cancer in Norfolk (EPIC-Norfolk) prospective population study. *Circulation* **116**: 2694–701.

Laughlin GA, Barrett-Connor E, Bergstrom J. (2008). Low testosterone and mortality in older men. *J Clin End Metab* **93**: 68–75.

Nieshlag E, Behre HE, Bouchard P, Corrales JJ, Jones TH, Stalla GK, Webb SM, Wu FCW. (2004). Testosterone replacement therapy: current trends and future directions. *Hum Reprod Update* **10**: 409–19.

Shores MM, Matsumoto AM, Sloan KL, Kivlahan DR. (2006). Low serum testosterone and mortality in male veterans. *Arch Intern Med* **166**: 1660–5.

Chapter 2

Clinical physiology of testosterone

T. Hugh Jones

Key points

- Adequate tissue androgenization is dependent on: the balance of testosterone synthesis and breakdown; the fraction of biologically active testosterone in the circulation and availability to the tissues; androgen receptor sensitivity; and non-genomic effects.
- Circulating testosterone is divided into three major fractions: free, albumin bound and sex hormone binding globulin bound. The free plus the albumin-bound testosterone constitutes the bioavailable testosterone.
- The CAG repeat androgen receptor polymorphism affects the sensitivity of the receptor and has clinical consequences.
- Some actions of testosterone are independent of the classical androgen receptor, which mediates effects through non-genomic mechanisms.
- Testosterone levels are affected adversely by age and obesity.

2.1 Introduction

Testosterone is mainly synthesized and secreted by the testes. The testes produce between 5 and 7 mg/day accounting for approximately 95% of the adult male's production. The remaining testosterone is produced by the zona reticularis of the adrenal cortex.

Testosterone release has a circadian rhythm with circulating levels peaking between 06.00 and 08.00 h and reaching a nadir between 18.00 and 20.00 h (see Figure 3.1, Chapter 3). Testosterone secretion also has a circannual rhythm with levels being highest in the late summer/late autumn and lowest at the end of winter/early spring.

The major biological actions of testosterone include the development and maintenance of secondary sexual characteristics as well as direct effects on several vital organs, body composition, and behaviour. There is now convincing evidence that testosterone has important metabolic and vascular effects.

The degree of androgenization is a state of balance between testosterone production and breakdown, the sensitivity of the androgen receptor, the presence of androgen receptor co-factors, the proportion of biologically active fraction of testosterone, and the effects of testosterone not mediated through the classical androgen receptor, including non-genomic actions. Elements that affect these parameters, will be discussed with respect to their clinical implications.

2.2 **Testosterone in the circulation**

There are three major fractions of testosterone in serum. The greatest proportion (50–80%) of testosterone is bound to sex hormone binding globulin (SHBG); 20–50% is bound to albumin, with 2–3% being free (unbound) (Figure 2.1). Testosterone also binds to other proteins, for example, cortisol-binding globulin, although the amount is very small and not of clinical significance. Free testosterone is rapidly metabolized by the liver and only has a short half-life of approximately 10 min.

Testosterone binds strongly to SHBG and slowly dissociates from the carrier protein. SHBG-bound testosterone is thus considered not to be readily available to the tissues although SHBG *per se* may have biological role. Free testosterone is rapidly metabolized so SHBG-bound testosterone may function as a circulating store of the hormone in men. The half-life of free testosterone is only 10 min, which demonstrates the importance of carrier protein binding and the continual synthesis and secretion of the hormone. Rodents, however, do not possess SHBG and this suggests there may be other explanations. Testosterone weakly binds to albumin and easily dissociates to become accessible for biological actions.

The free, coupled with the albumin-bound, testosterone is considered to be the biologically active or bioavailable testosterone. This is supported by studies that have shown close correlations of bioavailable testosterone with biological androgenic end-points, such as bone turnover, muscle strength, cardiac ischaemia, and quality of erections.

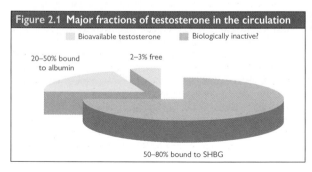

Figure 2.1 Major fractions of testosterone in the circulation

Bioavailable testosterone   Biologically inactive?

20–50% bound to albumin   2–3% free

50–80% bound to SHBG

2.3 **Sex hormone binding globulin**

SHBG is mainly synthesized in the liver, although some other tissues such as prostate can produce small amounts. SHBG is a large glycoprotein that forms homodimers and possesses two testosterone-binding sites. It has previously been suggested that SHBG is a carrier protein, stores testosterone in the circulation and when the hormone is bound it is inactive; however, recent evidence implies that SHBG bound testosterone may have specific effects other than testosterone storage. SHBG binds to an endocytic receptor (megalin) on the cell membrane and is then internalized into the cell. SHBG levels and SHBG polymorphisms are positively associated with bone mineral density suggesting an active role of this protein.

The circulating level of SHBG can be affected by several important clinical factors. Oestrogens stimulate SHBG synthesis, and levels also rise with age. Production is inhibited by obesity and clinical conditions associated with insulin resistance, such as the metabolic syndrome and type 2 diabetes. Evidence suggests that insulin is a potent inhibitor of hepatic SHBG production.

SHBG is an important marker of insulin resistance and several studies have shown that it is an independent predictor of the subsequent development of metabolic syndrome and type 2 diabetes. More recently it has been shown that atorvastatin and not simvastatin therapy is associated with lower SHBG levels in men with type 2 diabetes. If SHBG levels are affected by these conditions then this in turn will directly affect the value of total testosterone. Evidence suggests however, that through a homeostatic mechanism, values of bioavailable testosterone and free testosterone may be unaffected; for example, in men on statin therapy.

However, if there are profound effects on SHBG levels then the SHBG carrier store of testosterone may be sufficiently reduced to, in turn, result in lower levels of bioavailable and free testosterone. In ageing, the rise in SHBG and associated maintenance of total testosterone values may mask low levels of bioavailable and free testosterone.

2.4 **Testosterone synthesis**

Testosterone is synthesized from cholesterol in the Leydig cells of the testes. The source of cholesterol is either from local synthesis within the Leydig cell or from the circulation by receptor-mediated endocytosis of low-density lipoprotein (LDL). The conversion of cholesterol to pregnenolone is the rate-limiting reaction of testosterone synthesis. Luteinizing hormone (LH) regulates the rate of this reaction and therefore controls the overall rate of testosterone production. The pathway of testosterone biosynthesis and metabolism is shown in Figure 2.2.

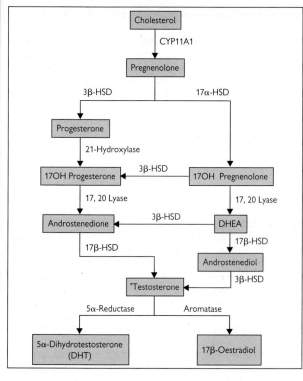

Figure 2.2 Pathway of testosterone synthesis and metabolism (CYP11A1=cholesterol side chain cleavage mitochondrial P450 enzyme, HSD=hydroxysteroid dehydrogenase, DHEA = dehydroepiandrosterone).
* Testosterone is also broken down to form inactive metabolites.

2.5 **Testosterone metabolism**

Testosterone is metabolized either to active or inactive metabolites.

2.5.1 **Active metabolites**

Testosterone is converted to 17β-oestradiol via the enzyme aromatase. Aromatase has its highest activity in adipose tissue, particularly visceral fat. The greater the volume of fat the greater the production of 17β-oestradiol. Other sites of aromatase activity are the testes, prostate, and bone.

Testosterone is converted to 5α-dihydrotestosterone (DHT) by 5α-reductase. The proportion of testosterone converted to oestradiol or DHT is likely to depend on the individual and tissue type. For example, testosterone and DHT are broken down by the liver and the resultant metabolites excreted by the kidneys.

The relative production of DHT and oestradiol varies between different tissues. For example, the production of DHT is much higher in the prostate and oestradiol is higher in bone.

2.5.2 **Inactive metabolites**

Testosterone and other androgens, including DHT, are inactivated by the liver by reduction, oxidation, hydroxylation and then conjugation with glucoronic acid, or sulphation. The metabolites are then excreted by the kidneys.

2.6 **Regulation of testosterone synthesis and secretion**

Gonadal function is dependent on the pulsatile secretion of both LH and follicle-stimulating hormone (FSH) from the anterior pituitary gland. Testosterone exerts a negative feedback upon the hypothalamus and pituitary inhibiting the secretion and pulsatility of LH release. The major action of LH is on the Leydig cells stimulating testosterone synthesis and secretion. LH stimulates the release of testosterone by the activation of cyclic adenosine monophosphate (cAMP). FSH acts primarily on the Sertoli cells and is involved in spermatogenesis. The release of FSH is mainly regulated by the negative feedback of inhibin that is secreted by the Sertoli cells.

2.6.1 **Hypothalamic–pituitary axis**

Gonadotrophin-releasing hormone (GnRH) is the major hypothalamic releasing factor that controls the secretion of LH and FSH from the gonadotrophs of the anterior pituitary (Figure 2.3). The hypothalamic release of GnRH is pulsatile with the amplitude and frequency of the pulse being critical for the stimulation of an LH pulse. Continuous exposure of the gonadotroph to GnRH results in desensitization of the GnRH receptor. This principle is used in the suppression of gonadotrophin secretion from the pituitary by GnRH analogue therapy for prostatic carcinoma. FSH pulses are more difficult to identify because of lower pulse amplitude and longer half-life.

Prolactin inhibits hypothalamic GnRH release. This is clinically relevant as hyperprolactinaemia suppresses the hypothalamic–pituitary–testicular axis, which results in hypogonadotrophic hypogonadism.

Figure 2.3 Regulation of the Hypothalamic-Pituitary–Testicular Axis

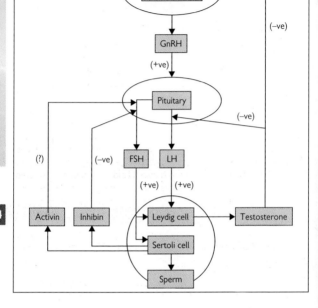

2.6.2 **Actions of gonadotrophins**

LH mediates its action on the testis through the LH receptor. LH rapidly stimulates testosterone secretion by increasing intracellular cAMP and intracellular calcium levels. LH enhances testosterone biosynthesis by several different mechanisms. The biochemical pathway of testosterone synthesis from cholesterol is described in Figure 2.2. The LH receptor can also be stimulated by human chorionic gonadotrophin (hCG). Although hCG is not produced in the male it has LH-like bioactivity and can be used to pharmacologically stimulate testosterone synthesis and release in men with hypothalamic–pituitary failure. Insulin-like growth factor-1 produced within the testis augments LH and hCG stimulatory effects on testosterone production in the Leydig cell. Glucocorticoids suppress testosterone production, whereas thyroid hormones stimulate the Leydig cell.

FSH acts primarily on the Sertoli cells and is involved in the initiation and maintenance of spermatogenesis. FSH also stimulates the synthesis and release of two hormones, inhibin and activin, from the Sertoli cells. Inhibin negatively feeds back on the hypothalamic–pituitary axis to specifically inhibit FSH release. There is no effect on LH secretion. The biological role of FSH-stimulated activin release is not known.

2.6.3 Inflammatory cytokines

Pro-inflammatory cytokines, which include interleukin (IL)-1, IL-6, tumour necrosis factor α (TNF-α), and interferons, are all known to inhibit the hypothalamic–pituitary–testicular axis. These cytokines have inhibitory effects at all levels of the axis. The suppressive effect is most profound in the presence of infection, inflammation, and infarction and after trauma, including surgery. Testosterone levels can fall as low as 2 nmol/l so assessment of androgen status is inappropriate under these conditions. Hypotestosteronaemia can lead to a reduced libido, which may be part of an evolutionary species protection system preventing sick individuals from procreation and thus favouring survival of the fittest. This would also explain the reduced libido commonly associated with common viral illnesses. Whether or not the loss of the anabolic effects of testosterone impairs recovery from trauma infection, inflammation or infarction is not known.

2.7 Androgen receptor sensitivity

2.7.1 The androgen receptor

The androgen receptor gene is situated on the long arm of the X chromosome (Xq11–12) and encodes for a protein of 910 amino acids. The male X chromosome and hence the androgen receptor is inherited from the mother. The androgen receptor belongs to a family of steroid and thyroid hormone receptors. The receptor gene consists of eight exons of which three main domains are involved in its biological function (Figure 2.4). Exon 1 comprises binding sites for co-activators. Exons 2 and 3 have two 'zinc' fingers that bind to androgen-sensitive genes. Exons 4–8 are involved with androgen binding.

Exon 1 is the site of a CAG repeat polymorphism that encodes for a polyglutamine stretch, which in turn affects androgen receptor sensitivity. The polymorphism affects the ability of two co-activator proteins (ARA24, p160) to bind, reducing receptor sensitivity. In the normal population the number of CAG repeats varies between 9 and 35. The greater the number of CAG repeats the less sensitive the receptor. The effect of the polymorphism may differ between tissues, as although the co-activators are ubiquitous they are not uniformly expressed.

There is also a GGC repeat polymorphism in Exon 1 which encodes for a polyglycine stretch. Whether or not this has clinical importance is under investigation.

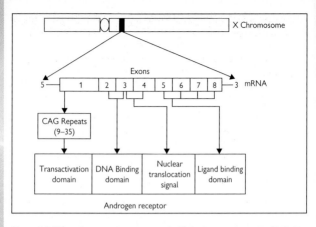

Figure 2.4 The androgen receptor gene on the X chromosome in section Xq11–12, which encodes for eight exons. The androgen receptor has four main functional domains: (1) The transactivation domain, which in the inactive state binds chaperone proteins that optimize ligand affinity, and in the active state binds co-activator proteins, which enhance ligand binding. (2) DNA binding domain with two zinc fingers. (3) Nuclear translocation signal to transport the active receptor from the cytosol to the nucleus. (4) Ligand binding domain.

Chaperone proteins, heat shock proteins (Hsp) Hsp 70, Hsp 90, p23 and co-chaperones Hsp 40 and Hop bind to the transactivation domain to maintain the optimal conformation necessary to bind the androgen to the receptor. Androgen binding to the receptor induces a conformational change in the protein that promotes dimerization of two androgen receptors, which then translocate to the nucleus. This dimerization increases the ability of the receptor to bind to androgen response elements on androgen-sensitive genes. The androgen receptor then mediates its effects through genomic mechanisms. Co-activator proteins regulate activation of transcription on binding of the androgen receptor to the androgen response elements.

2.7.2 **CAG repeat polymorphism**

Studies of healthy male populations have shown an important relationship between the length of the CAG repeat and biological and clinical parameters (Table 2.1). Greater androgen receptor sensitivity (low CAG repeat numbers) have been found to be associated with higher sperm concentration, increased bone mineral density and prostate size, benign prostatic hyperplasia, and an increased risk of prostate carcinoma. There is a greater chance of a man having surgery for benign prostatic hypertrophy if the CAG repeat length is 19 or less compared with 25 or greater. These men also are more likely to have low high-density lipoprotein cholesterol levels; however, other studies have found that higher circulating testosterone levels are associated

Table 2.1 Effect of CAG repeat length on biological and medical parameters

CAG repeat number	
Low (high receptor sensitivity)	**High (low receptor sensitivity)**
Healthy men	
↑ Prostate size	↑ BMI
↑ Penile length	↑ Leptin
↑ Risk of BPH	↑ Fasting insulin
↑ Risk prostate cancer	↑ Body fat content
↑ Sperm count	↑ HDL-cholesterol
↑ BMD	↓ BMD
↑ Risk of conduct disorders	↑ Risk of depression
↑ Risk of ADH	↑ LH
↑ Risk of drug abuse	
↑ Risk of pathological gambling	
Klinefelter's Syndrome	
Stable partnership	↑ Gynaecomastia
Profession with high standard of education	↓ Testes size
↑ Height	
↓ Arm span: height ratio	
↓ BMD	
After TRT	
↑ Hb	
↑ Prostate growth	
↑ LH suppression	
BPH=Benign prostatic hypertrophy, ADH=Attention deficit hyperactivity disorder, Hb=Haemoglobin	

with higher high-density lipoprotein cholesterol. Men with less sensitive androgen receptors were found to be associated with higher body fat content, body mass index, leptin and insulin levels. There are no clear associations of androgen receptor sensitivity with mood; however, one study reported a higher incidence of drug abuse and pathological gambling with short CAG repeats.

The Massachusetts Male Aging study has found that total and free testosterone levels are positively correlated with CAG repeat number, although this has not been confirmed in other studies. LH levels are found to be higher in the top quartile of CAG repeat length suggesting that the hypothalamic–pituitary production of LH compensates for the more insensitive receptor by stimulating greater synthesis and release of testosterone.

The mean CAG repeat length differs between ethnic groups: in Afro-Caribbeans it is 18–20, Caucasians 21–22, and East Asians 22–23. Interestingly, this may explain the higher rate of prostate cancer in the Afro-Caribbean population.

In men with Klinefelter's Syndrome CAG repeats predicted phenotypic features (Table 2.1). Those patients with longer repeats were more likely to have gynaecomastia, smaller testicular size, lower bone mineral density, were taller (reduced arm span to height ratio), with higher body mass index and oestradiol levels. Klinefelter men with shorter repeats were also more likely to have a partner with a stable relationship and more likely to present for investigation of infertility. Men with shorter repeats were more likely to be highly skilled professionals. Furthermore, Klinefelter men with shorter repeats were more likely to be diagnosed later in life. Testosterone substitution led to a greater prostate growth and increase in haemoglobin levels in men with shorter CAG repeats.

Kennedy's Syndrome is a rare condition where expansion of the CAG repeat number to greater than normal is associated with a neurodegenerative disorder that is characterized by progressive neuromuscular weakness as a result of motor neuron loss in the spinal cord and brain stem. The neurological symptoms usually first occur in the third to fifth decade of life. This condition is associated with raised gonadotrophin levels, gynaecomastia, testicular atrophy, impaired spermatogenesis, and diabetes.

2.8 Non-genomic actions of testosterone

It has become increasingly recognized that steroid hormones mediate some of their biological effects through mechanisms that are independent of the genomically acting classic steroid receptors. Testosterone and other androgens have rapid effects occurring within 2–3 min. The fastest known genomic effect is approximately 40 min, so by definition these effects are not being mediated genomically via the classic androgen receptor.

Studies have shown that testosterone has direct effects at the cell membrane. These include inhibition of calcium fluxes in macrophages, T cells (which do not possess androgen receptors), and vascular smooth muscle cells. In vascular smooth muscle cells in cell culture testosterone inhibits L-calcium channels by binding at the same site as nifedipine (see Chapter 12). Testosterone inhibits potassium efflux in vascular smooth muscle cells, stimulates gonadotrophin release from the pituitary, and prostate-specific antigen release by prostate cells through non-genomic mechanisms. Testosterone has also been found to stimulate second messenger systems, for example, MAP kinase.

2.9 **Biological actions of testosterone and its metabolites**

The effects of testosterone are either mediated directly through testosterone or its two major active metabolites, DHT and 17β-oestradiol. Sexual differentiation in the embryo, during puberty, and maintenance of virilization is mainly dependent on a combination of effects of testosterone and DHT. DHT, which also mediates its effects through the androgen receptor, plays a greater part in the development of deepening of the voice, increasing sebum production, and enlargement of the external genitalia, including penile length. The importance of DHT is demonstrated by the finding that reduced or absent function of 5α reductase is associated with the micropenis.

The conversion of testosterone to DHT in the prostate is essential for its growth and development. The concentration of DHT in the prostate is 10 times higher than testosterone. A genetic defect in 5α-reductase results in the failure of prostate development even in the presence of normal prostatic testosterone levels. The clinical importance of this is underlined by the effective use of finasteride (a 5α-reductase inhibitor) in the management of benign prostatic hypertrophy.

The effects of the testosterone and DHT are highly dependent on the topographical site. For example, beard growth is dependent on testosterone, whereas axillary and pubic hair growth is DHT dependent. Furthermore, DHT inhibits scalp hair growth leading to male pattern baldness in some men. Whether or not a man develops baldness may be related to the relative activities of 5α-reductase and aromatase activity within the scalp.

Muscle growth and strength is linked to testosterone and not DHT. This is demonstrated by the lack of effect of finasteride on muscle parameters. Testosterone enhances haematopoiesis by two mechanisms, first by stimulating renal and extra-renal erythropoietin production and secondly by a direct effect on the bone marrow. Oestrogen production in the male is essential to maintain bone integrity. Men with aromatase deficiency all develop osteoporosis. Oestradiol also plays an important part in stimulating epiphyseal closure.

There is increasing evidence that testosterone has effects on metabolism: enhancing insulin sensitivity and glucose tolerance, stimulating expression of mitochondrial genes involved in oxidative phosphorylation and mitochondrial function. Testosterone is also associated with lipid metabolism, although the exact mechanisms by which testosterone is associated with lower cholesterol and higher high-density lipoprotein cholesterol levels has not as yet been elucidated. There is evidence from animal studies that oestradiol formed from testosterone stimulates HDL cholesterol levels. Testosterone has been shown to act as a vasodilator, which is endothelial independent, directly acting on vascular smooth muscle cells. In addition oestradiol is also known to be a vasodilator mediating its effects via nitric oxide.

Testosterone has important psychotropic actions on the brain, which include enhancing drive, motivation, improving mood and libido. Testosterone also improves cognitive functions such as visual–spatial skills, short-term memory, and mathematical ability. Testosterone status is negatively correlated with verbal fluency. These factors can influence social and cultural issues.

Erectile dysfunction is associated with testosterone deficiency. In animal studies, testosterone deficiency is associated with loss of elastic fibres, which are replaced by collagen in the tunica albuginea, nerve sheaths and vascular smooth muscle cells. Furthermore, adipocytes become apparent between the tunica albuginea and the corpus cavernosum. This evidence suggests that testosterone is important in maintaining a normal penile architecture. Evidence shows that the normal action of nitric oxide, which is the main agent that produces the erection, is androgen dependent.

FSH is essential in the initiation of spermatogenesis at puberty. Once spermatogenesis has been established it can be maintained in the absence of FSH. LH stimulation of testosterone production, however, is important in the maintenance of adequate spermatogenesis. Spermatogenesis does require sufficiently high levels of intratesticular testosterone.

2.10 **Age**

After the age of 40, testosterone levels fall by 1–2% per annum. The decline is attenuated and there is maintenance of the circadian rhythm when fitness is sustained. Studies have found that 7% of men between 40 and 60 years, 21% between 60 and 80 years, and 35% of men greater than 80 years of age have total testosterone concentrations of less than 12 nmol/l. Using assessment of total testosterone in older men is complicated by the age-related increase in SHBG, which can mask significantly lower levels of the biologically active fraction. The fall in testosterone production is caused by a combination of hypothalamic–pituitary and testicular failure. However, visceral obesity associated with aging is likely also to be a factor, which lowers testosterone levels. Late-onset hypogonadism and the effects of aging are discussed in more detail in Chapter 6.

2.11 **Obesity**

Aromatase concentration and activity is proportional to the amount of adipose tissue. It has a greater activity in visceral than subcutaneous fat.

Therefore, the degree of obesity is directly proportional to the metabolism of testosterone to oestradiol. The homeostatic response of the hypothalamic–pituitary–testicular axis to the fall in testosterone is impaired by the inhibitory effects of the higher oestradiol levels, leptin resistance, and the suppressive actions of pro-inflammatory adipocytokines. Testosterone inhibits adipocyte lipoprotein lipase. A reduction in testosterone would lead to increased activity of the enzyme thus promoting triglyceride uptake and adipocyte proliferation. This is the basis of the Hypogonadal–Obesity–Adipocytokine cycle hypothesis described in more detail in Chapter 11.

Key references

Kaufman JM, Vermeulen A. (2005). The decline in androgen levels in elderly men and its clinical implications. *Endocr Rev* **26**: 833–76.

Zitzmann M. (2007). Mechanisms of disease: pharmacogenetics of testosterone therapy in hypogonadal men. *Nat Clin Pract Urol* **4**: 161–6.

Zitzmann M, Nieschlag E. (2003). The CAG repeat polymorphism within the androgen receptor gene and maleness. *Int J Androl* **76**: 76–83.

Chapter 3

Diagnosis of hypogonadism: symptoms, signs, tests, and guidelines

T. Hugh Jones

> ### Key points
>
> - Hypogonadism is a clinical syndrome complex that comprises symptoms ± signs as well as biochemical evidence of testosterone deficiency.
> - The clinical presentation of hypogonadism depends on the age of onset and whether or not it is pre- or post-puberty.
> - Symptoms of hypogonadism especially in older men are non-specific.
> - The measurement of morning total testosterone is a good predictor of hypogonadism, except in borderline cases where free or bioavailable testosterone assessment can be more sensitive.
> - Published guidelines have aided clinicians in the diagnosis of hypogonadism especially in the interpretation of testosterone levels.

3.1 Diagnosis of hypogonadism

Hypogonadism is a clinical syndrome complex that comprises symptoms ± signs as well as biochemical evidence of testosterone deficiency. The clinical diagnosis of hypogonadism can be difficult in a significant proportion of subjects because the symptoms of testosterone deficiency are non-specific and the biochemical tests not easy to interpret. Furthermore, guidelines for the diagnosis of hypogonadism can vary between international and national societies. Some countries indeed have no guidelines. The normal ranges of testosterone used in clinical laboratories are based on normal ranges of healthy young men. These ranges, especially the lower limits, can also vary between countries and laboratories.

The ultimate decision on the diagnosis of hypogonadism should be made by an experienced clinician in the field, as once treatment is commenced the patient usually remains on therapy for many years. It is, however, important that doctors in all specialities, including primary care, are aware of the symptoms, tests, guidelines, and associations of testosterone deficiency with other medical conditions. Once initial tests suggest a diagnosis of hypogonadism the patient needs to be referred to an appropriate specialist for confirmation of the diagnosis, investigation of the underlying cause, initiation and monitoring of therapy.

3.2 **Symptoms**

The presentation of hypogonadism will depend on whether the onset was pre-pubertal or post-pubertal.

3.2.1 **Pre-pubertal onset**

The commonest presenting symptom is that of failure to enter puberty. This is manifested by lack of development of secondary sexual characteristics. These mainly comprise lack of secondary sexual hair, lack of development of the genitalia, eunoichoid body shape and failure of deepening of the voice. It is sometimes associated with gynaecomastia, a history of cryptorchidism, tall stature, or growth retardation.

The cause of delayed puberty is classified into constitutional delayed puberty and failure of puberty as a result of specific conditions, which include inheritable and acquired disorders. The specific conditions that may present with failure of puberty will be discussed in Chapters 4 and 5. A detailed management of delayed puberty will be included in Chapter 9.

3.2.2 **Post-pubertal onset**

The presenting symptoms particularly in older men are variable. Many men will not volunteer information regarding their sex drive or inability to attain an erection. The clinic situation is a dynamic one and will depend on the clinical skills of the doctor to obtain a full medical history. The presence of the patient's wife or partner at the consultation sometimes helps but in certain circumstances can hinder it. In many instances the wife or partner has instigated the man to seek medical advice.

The most well recognized symptom of hypogonadism is reduced or loss of libido. This symptom in particular can lead to breakdown of relationships and marriages. It also results in loss of self-esteem and confidence. A fall in libido can, however, be commonly associated with other medical conditions, which include depression, anxiety, and acute and chronic disease states.

Testosterone deficiency is also associated with a reduction in the strength of erection and loss of early morning erections. Vascular disease, hypertension, autonomic neuropathy, drugs (e.g. beta-blockers) and psychogenic disorders can all cause erectile dysfunction in addition to hypogonadism. The coexistence of testosterone deficiency with other causes of erectile dysfunction increases the severity. It is recommended that testosterone levels should be assessed in all men presenting with erectile dysfunction. The importance of normal androgen status in achieving an erection has been demonstrated in men who fail to respond to PDE5 inhibitors, such as sildenafil, who have a higher incidence of testosterone deficiency than responders. Testosterone substitution converts 60% of sildenafil non-responders to responders.

Fatigue is a common symptom of hypogonadism. The fatigue can be profound and equivalent to that found in patients presenting with hypothyroidism. The clinical history usually reveals a type of fatigue consistent with an organic rather than psychological cause. The salient features of this type of fatigue, unless there is a psychological component, are that the individual usually sleeps well and on waking feels refreshed compared with going to bed. As the day progresses he feels gradually more and more tired and lethargic. There may also be a tendency to fall asleep during the day particularly after meals; classically after the evening meal. This symptom has to be taken in context, as in some cultures this is the acceptable norm.

Another symptom is where there is a reduced ability to undertake physical tasks that require endurance; for example, gardening or distance walking. This loss of physical endurance is consistent with reduced muscle strength and also motivation and mood. Older men with testosterone deficiency tend to become frailer. This frailty increases the risk of falls and if there is associated osteopenia or osteoporosis this can potentially lead to fractures. Hypogonadal men may therefore present to the accident and emergency, orthopaedic, or rheumatology departments.

Mood disturbance is another important symptom. Hypogonadal men have a tendency to be more depressed, irritable, and have poor concentration. Mood swings can manifest themselves in the individual becoming grumpy and sometimes more aggressive. These frustrations may be due in part to their reduced ability to have sexual intercourse and also as a result of direct effects on the brain. Some men, however, appear to be more placid. Testosterone deficiency is also associated with more negative than positive thoughts. The specific symptoms, which a person manifests, may be related to their individual psyche prior to developing hypogonadism.

Men with testosterone deficiency, who have reduced visuospatial cognitive function can improve with testosterone substitution. This can be associated with impaired visual and verbal memory.

Excessive sweating and hot flushes can occur in some men but generally this is not a common symptom.

Hypogonadotrophic hypogonadism is invariably associated with a reduced (oligospermia) or absent (azospermia) sperm count. In primary testicular failure the presence of oligospermia or azospermia will depend on the aetiology and severity of the underlying disorder. The quality of the morphology and motility of sperm may also be impaired in primary and secondary hypogonadism.

3.3 Signs

The emphasis on the different clinical signs of testosterone deficiency varies according to the age of presentation. Males presenting with failure of puberty (which can be at any age) may have a eunuchoid body habitus with gynaecomastia and female distribution of body fat. They may be tall and there may be a greater ratio of arm span to height. This occurs, as there is failure of the epiphyseal plates to close resulting in faster and continued long bone growth.

Facial features are boyish with lack of facial hair, and maintenance of the frontal hairline. The skin can be pale, dry and there is a lack of acne. Muscles are underdeveloped and strength reduced. The voice may not be broken and can be high pitched. There is invariably a lack of secondary sexual body hair. Some pubic hair may be present but in a characteristic female distribution and may be sparse. The genitalia are underdeveloped with a small penis (normal adult flaccid length is approximately 6 cm). Testicular size is assessed using the Prader orchiometer. Normal testicular size varies between 12 and 25 ml with a mean length of 4.6 cm (range 3.5–5.5 cm). If there is complete or near complete testosterone deficiency as a result of hypogonadotrophic hypogonadism the testes are very small (less than 4 ml). In the presence of gonadotrophins, provided there is no state of testosterone resistance, then testicular size can be normal. The scrotal skin may be wrinkled and lack pigmentation.

Hypogonadism may be a manifestation of hypopituitarism or coexist with other medical conditions. Therefore, the practitioner needs to be aware of related disorders, such as Cushing's disease, craniopharyngioma and chronic diseases, which may present with hypogonadism (these conditions are dealt with in Chapter 5).

Post-pubertal hypogonadism may not be associated with any overt clinical signs. The presence of signs will depend on the degree and duration of testosterone deficiency. The classical features are fine wrinkling of the facial skin especially around the mouth and eyes, and maintenance of the frontal hairline. Hypogonadism may be associated with truncal, particularly visceral obesity and muscle atrophy, and reduced strength. There may be loss of height and other features of osteoporosis such as kyphoscoliosis. Again it is imperative to undertake a **full** examination for signs of related causes of hypogonadism (see Chapters 4 and 5). Abdominal examination, for example, may reveal hepatomegaly (e.g. in haemochromatosis) and splenomegaly (e.g. in lymphoma), which may both be associated with presentation of hypopituitarism.

3.4 Questionnaires

There are two questionnaires that are validated and available as a diagnostic aid in older men. These questionnaires should not be used in isolation as they have low specificity; however, they have reasonably high sensitivity in association with a low serum testosterone.

3.4.1 ADAM

The St Louis University Androgen Deficiency in Aging Males (ADAM) questionnaire is a simple 10-question yes/no answer format (Table 3.1). The questionnaire is positive if there are positive answers to either questions 1 or 7, or three other questions. The ADAM questionnaire has an 88% sensitivity but <60% specificity. This questionnaire can be useful in the initial consultation as sometimes the patient may not volunteer sexual symptoms due to embarrassment but may readily fill out the form.

Table 3.1 **ADAM Questionnaire. A positive score consistent with hypogonadism is a yes response to either question 1 or 7 or three other affirmative answers**

	Yes	No
Do you have a decrease in libido (sex drive)?		
Do you have a lack of energy?		
Do you have a decrease in strength and/or endurance?		
Have you lost height?		
Have you noticed a decreased enjoyment of life?		
Are you sad and/or grumpy?		
Are your erections less strong?		
Have you noticed a recent deterioration in your ability to play sports?		
Are you falling asleep after dinner?		
Has there been a recent deterioration in your work performance?		

3.4.2 **AMS**

The Aging Males' Symptoms (AMS) rating scale questionnaire is more detailed (Table 3.2). The questionnaire is divided into three domains: physical, somatic and psychological, including impairment of sexual performance. The main advantage is that the patient can provide degrees of symptoms on a scale. The disadvantage is that it is more complicated. The severity of symptoms correlates well with an estimate

Table 3.2 The Aging Males' Symptom (AMS) Scale

AMS Questionnaire

Which of the following symptoms apply to you at this time? Please, mark the appropriate box for each symptom. For symptoms that do not apply, please mark 'none'.

Symptoms:	none	mild	moderate	severe	extremely severe
Score =	1	2	3	4	5
1. **Decline in your feeling of general well-being** (general state of health, subjective feeling)	☐	☐	☐	☐	☐
2. **Joint pain and muscular ache** (lower back pain, joint pain, pain in a limb, general back ache)	☐	☐	☐	☐	☐
3. **Excessive sweating** (unexpected/sudden episodes of sweating, hot flushes independent of strain)	☐	☐	☐	☐	☐
4. **Sleep problems** (difficulty in falling asleep, difficulty in sleeping through, waking up early and feeling tired, poor sleep, sleeplessness)	☐	☐	☐	☐	☐
5. **Increased need for sleep, often feeling tired**	☐	☐	☐	☐	☐
6. **Irritability** (feeling aggressive, easily upset about little things, moody)	☐	☐	☐	☐	☐
7. **Nervousness** (inner tension, restlessness, feeling fidgety)	☐	☐	☐	☐	☐
8. **Anxiety** (feeling panicky)	☐	☐	☐	☐	☐
9. **Physical exhaustion/lacking vitality** (general decrease in performance, reduced activity, lacking interest in leisure activities, feeling of getting less done, of achieving less, of having to force oneself to undertake activities)	☐	☐	☐	☐	☐
10. **Decrease in muscular strength** (feeling of weakness)	☐	☐	☐	☐	☐
11. **Depressive mood** (feeling down, sad, on the verge of tears, lack of drive, mood swings, feeling nothing is of any use)	☐	☐	☐	☐	☐
12. **Feeling that you have passed your peak**	☐	☐	☐	☐	☐
13. **Feeling burnt out, having hit rock-bottom**	☐	☐	☐	☐	☐
14. **Decrease in beard growth**	☐	☐	☐	☐	☐
15. **Decrease in ability/frequency to perform sexually**	☐	☐	☐	☐	☐
16. **Decrease in the number of morning erections**	☐	☐	☐	☐	☐
17. **Decrease in sexual desire/libido** (lacking pleasure in sex, lacking desire for sexual intercourse)	☐	☐	☐	☐	☐

Have you got any other major symptoms? Yes ····· ☐   No ····· ☐
If Yes, please describe: _ _ _ _ _ _ _ _ _ _ _ _ _ _ _ _ _ _ .

_ _

THANK YOU VERY MUCH FOR YOUR COOPERATION

of testosterone deficiency by an experienced clinician. There are no clear cut-off score values diagnostic of hypogonadism. It is most useful, however, in documenting and comparing the scores before and after testosterone replacement therapy to assess the clinical response.

These questionnaires are useful but should only be used as an adjunct to making the diagnosis of hypogonadism. There is no questionnaire specifically designed to monitor the efficacy of testosterone replacement therapy.

3.5 Guidelines – symptoms and signs

The Endocrine Society of the USA published Clinical Practice Guidelines for Testosterone Therapy in Adult Men with Androgen Deficiency Syndromes in 2006. The committee recommended dividing hypogonadal symptoms and signs into two groups (Table 3.3): (1) symptoms and signs suggestive of androgen deficiency in which physicians should measure serum testosterone levels (Table 3.3A), (2) other symptoms and signs associated with androgen deficiency but less specific (Table 3.3B) (if these symptoms and signs occur in conjunction with those of the first group testosterone levels should also be measured).

It is important and mandatory that the testosterone levels are assessed on more than one occasion, as up to one-third of men with low levels have normal levels when repeated.

Table 3.3 Endocrine Society's Clinical Guidelines classification of symptoms and signs of androgen deficiency	
A. Symptoms and signs suggestive of androgen deficiency	**B. Symptoms and signs associated with androgen deficiency that are less specific**
↓ Sexual desire (libido) and activity	↓ Energy, motivation, initiative, aggressiveness, self-confidence
↓ Spontaneous erections	Feeling sad or blue, depressed mood, dysthymia
Breast discomfort, gynaecomastia	Poor concentration and memory
Loss of axillary and pubic hair, ↓ shaving	Sleep disturbance, ↑ sleepiness
Very small or shrinking testes (especially <5 ml)	Mild anaemia (normochromic, normocytic)
Incomplete sexual development, eunuchoidism aspermia	↑ body fat, ↑ body mass index
Inability to father children, low or zero sperm counts	Diminished physical or work performance
Height loss, low trauma fracture, ↓ bone mineral density	
↓ muscle bulk and strength	
Hot flushes, sweats	

3.6 **Biochemical tests**

3.6.1 **Total testosterone**

Serum measurement of total testosterone is the most widely used screening test for hypogonadism. Venous blood should be taken before 11.00 h to avoid misdiagnosis as a result of the circadian rhythm giving lower testosterone levels later in the day. This rule should be adhered to in older as well as younger men (Figure 3.1). Testosterone levels should be assessed on at least two separate days and in some instances, where the tests are borderline on three or more occasions. Systemic illness such as intercurrent infections can lower testosterone levels and may be higher than baseline after sexual intercourse the night before.

There are no clear cut-offs of total testosterone values below which a symptomatic man can be confidently diagnosed as having hypogonadism. Clearly, in the presence of symptoms and signs and total testosterone levels consistently below 8 mmol/l there is little doubt that hypogonadism exists. Normal ranges of total testosterone are usually based on healthy young men. Normal ranges, particularly the lower limit, vary between laboratories and different commercial assays. Some concern regarding this has been raised by the Endocrine Society. Generally, however, the total testosterone assay is good enough to be able to distinguish between the eugonadal and

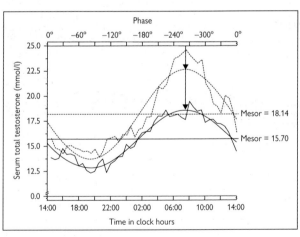

Figure 3.1 Cosinor-derived circadian rhythmometry (CHRONOLAB) for plasma total testosterone concentration in 10 young men (dotted line) and in eight middle-aged men, which included men into their seventh decade (solid line) showing the diurnal rhythm maintained in both groups of men. Reproduced with permission from Diver, MJ et al (2003). *Clinical Endocrinology* (Oxford) **58** (6): 141–150.

hypogonadal state. The difficulties arise in borderline levels and understanding the thresholds of total testosterone levels recommended by different guidelines.

Significant difficulties in using total testosterone to diagnose hypogonadism arise in conditions which affect levels of the sex hormone binding globulin (SHBG). As described below these include such common conditions as: diabetes, metabolic syndrome, obesity, ageing, smoking and statin therapy.

3.6.2 Sex hormone binding globulin

SHBG should be assayed with the second sample if the first total testosterone level is borderline and in men with conditions that may affect SHBG (Table 3.4). Assessment of SHBG is particularly important in older men, obesity, metabolic syndrome, and diabetes. The SHBG value can then be used in equations to calculate either the free or bioavailable testosterone level as described below.

3.6.3 Free testosterone

The only assay to measure free testosterone, which is acceptable, is by equilibrium dialysis. This is a time-consuming assay and is generally only found in research laboratories. It is therefore not amenable for routine clinical use. Measurement of free testosterone directly by immunoassay is unreliable, is still influenced by the level of SHBG, and is not recommended by international guidelines.

The best routine assessment of free testosterone, although not ideal, is mathematical calculation using the total testosterone and SHBG levels. However, there are several published equations that can give differing results. The Vermeulen Equation is the most commonly used as a calculator and is available on the website www.issam.ch/freetesto.htm. Ideally, the calculated free testosterone should be validated by the local laboratory.

Table 3.4 Factors which affect SHBG levels	
Increased SHBG	**Decreased SHBG**
Ageing	Insulin resistance
Thyrotoxicosis	Obesity
Acromegaly	Metabolic syndrome
Smoking	Type 2 diabetes
Cirrhosis of liver	Atorvastatin
Anticonvulsants	Hypothyroidism
HIV	Glucocorticoids
Rosiglitazone	Anabolic steroids
	Low albumin states, e.g. nephrotic syndrome

31

3.6.4 **Bioavailable testosterone**

Bioavailable testosterone can be assayed using the modified method of Tremblay and Dube using ammonium sulphate precipitation of SHBG. This is again a time-consuming assay and generally not suitable for routine clinical use. However, in the USA bioavailable testosterone can be measured by a commercial laboratory.

Mathematical formulae are also available to calculate the bioavailable testosterone using the total testosterone and the SHBG; one formula is available on the website www.him-link.com. Once again it is important to validate the equation in the local laboratory as there are differences between total testosterone and SHBG assays that may affect the calculated value.

3.6.5 **Gonadotrophins**

Elevated luteinizing hormone (LH) levels are consistent with a diagnosis of primary hypogonadism. LH levels below the normal range are usually consistent with secondary or hypogonadotrophic hypogonadism. Low levels of LH associated with low testosterone levels occur in states of acute injury (including surgery), infection, inflammation, or infarction (e.g. myocardial). These effects are usually transient and recover once the physical insult has resolved.

Normal levels of LH may occur in hypogonadism associated with obesity or ageing. The nomenclature for classification is not clear and has been considered as hypogonadotrophic hypogonadism, mixed hypogonadism, or normogonadotrophic hypogonadism. Ageing is most likely a combination of hypothalamic–pituitary failure as well as testicular failure, and, therefore, could be classified as mixed hypogonadism. Hypogonadism is associated with visceral adiposity causing increased testosterone metabolism and impaired hypothalamic–pituitary axis response to the testosterone deficiency as a result of suppression of the axis by adipocytokines, leptin resistance, and increased oestradiol levels.

Elevated follicle-stimulating hormone (FSH) levels indicate Sertoli cell failure. Low FSH is consistent with hypopituitarism. Ageing men may have raised follicle-stimulating hormone with normal LH.

3.6.6 **Prolactin**

Prolactin levels should be measured in hypogonadism associated with low or low normal LH. Hyperprolactinaemia may present as hypogonadism. The causes of hyperprolactinaemia are discussed in Chapter 5.

3.7 **Guidelines – testosterone levels**

3.7.1 **Endocrine Society (USA) 2006**

The Endocrine Society (USA) Guidelines state the following:

> *The threshold testosterone levels below which symptoms of androgen deficiency and adverse health outcomes occur is not known and may be age dependent. Furthermore, the testosterone concentration below which testosterone administration improves outcome is unknown and may vary among individuals and among target organs. Therefore, the available evidence does not support use of an arbitrary threshold for testosterone levels below which clinical androgen deficiency occurs and that confirms the diagnosis of hypogonadism in all patients.*

These guidelines however, have advised a cut-off for total testosterone, which is 10.4 nmol/l (300 ng/dl). It has been shown in two studies that there are benefits in testosterone replacement therapy for men below this level. First, testosterone substitution improves spinal bone mineral density in men only with a baseline total testosterone less than 10.4 nmol/l. A second study found an identical level where this level of testosterone maintained fat-free mass.

3.7.2 **ISA, ISSAM, and EAU Recommendations for Late-onset Hypogonadism 2006**

The International Society for Andrology (ISA), the International Society for the Study of the Aging Male (ISSAM), and European Association of Urology (EAU) published 2006 recommendations for the investigation, treatment, and monitoring of late-onset hypogonadism. They stated the following:

> *There are no generally accepted lower limits of normal (total testosterone) and it is unclear whether geographically different thresholds depend on ethnic differences or on the physician's perception. There is, however, general agreement that total testosterone levels above 12 nmol/l (346 ng/dl) or free testosterone levels above 250 pmol/l (72 pg/ml) do not require substitution. Similarly, based on the data of younger men, there is a consensus that serum total testosterone levels below 8 nmol/l (231 ng/dl) or free testosterone below 180 pmol/l (52 pg/ml) require substitution. Since symptoms of testosterone deficiency become manifest between 12 and 8 nmol/l, trials of treatment can be considered in those in whom alternative causes of these symptoms have been excluded. (Since there are variations in the reagents and normal ranges among laboratories, the cut-off values given for serum testosterone and free testosterone may have to be adjusted depending on the reference values given by the laboratory.)*

3.8 **Symptoms and testosterone levels**

A recent study in older men (50–86 years) presenting to an andrology clinic has found that the prevalence of loss of libido or vigour, increased with testosterone levels below 15 nmol/l. Obesity was more prevalent below 12 nmol/l, and type 2 diabetes and depression below 10 nmol/l. Erectile dysfunction and hot flushes had a greater prevalence below 8 nmol/l. These findings are interesting but the authors do recommend that they should not be taken in isolation and that a broad holistic approach should be taken to the clinical assessment.

3.9 **Conclusions**

It is recognized that the diagnosis of hypogonadism is not straight-forward unless there are equivocally low testosterone levels associated with classical symptoms and signs. In an attempt to aid the physician recent guidelines have been published, although there are differences between them. A suggested algorithm, which takes into account these recommendations, is provided in Figure 3.2.

Hypogonadism is an underdiagnosed condition. There does need to be an increased awareness of the condition and its diagnosis. If symptoms are present then testosterone levels should be assessed. An experienced clinician should make the final diagnosis and decision to treat. As symptoms are non-specific and the biochemical tests can be difficult to interpret in borderline cases then a trial of testosterone replacement therapy of up to 3 months can be considered.

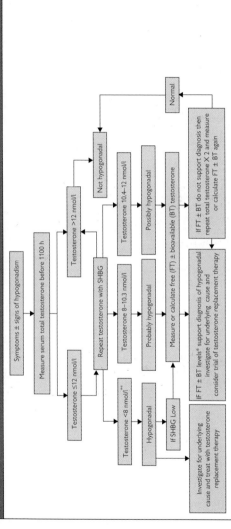

Figure 3.2 Suggested algorithm to assist clinicians in the diagnosis of hypogonadism

Suggested algorithm to assist clinicians in the diagnosis of hypogonadism. Symptoms of hypogonadism must be present; however, men with osteoporosis and low stress fractures could also be considered. * If SHBG is below the normal range measurement or calculation of FT ± BT is recommended. ** The levels of free and bioavailable testosterone at which men are considered to be hypogonadal should be validated locally but there are levels based on published evidence to guide the clinician as well. If a diagnosis of hypogonadism is considered then appropriate investigation for an underlying cause should be undertaken (see Chapters 4, 5, and 6). If the tests are suggestive, but not conclusive, a trial of testosterone replacement therapy of up to 3 months can be considered provided there are no contraindications.

Key references

Bhasin S, Cunningham GR, Hayes FJ et al. (2006). Testosterone therapy in adult men with androgen deficiency syndromes: an Endocrine Society Clinical Practice Guideline. *J Clin End Metab* **91**: 1995–2010.

Heinnemann LAJ, Zimmerman T, Vermeulen A et al. (2001). A new aging males' symptoms rating scale. *Aging Male* **2**: 105–14.

Morley JE, Charlton E, Patrick P et al. (2000). Validation of a screening questionnaire for androgen deficiency in aging males. *Metabolism* **49**: 1239–42.

Morris PD, Malkin CJ, Channer KS et al. (2004). A mathematical comparison of techniques to predict biologically active testosterone in a cohort of 1072 men. *Eur J Endocrinol* **151**: 241–9.

Nieschlag E, Behre HM, Bouchard P, et al. (2004). Testosterone replacement therapy: current trends and future directions. *Hum Reprod Update* **5**: 409–11.

Nieschlag E, Swerdloff R, Behre HM et al. (2006). Investigation, treatment and monitoring of late-onset hypogonadism in males: ISA, ISSAM and EAU recommendations. *J Androl* **27**: 135–7.

Ronde W, van der Schouw YT, Pols HAP et al. (2006). Calculation of bioavailable and free testosterone in men: a comparison of 5 published algorithms. *Clin Chem* **52**: 1777–84.

Rosner W, Auchus RJ, Azziz R et al. (2007). Position statement: utility, limitations, and pitfalls in measuring testosterone: an Endocrine Society position statement. *J Clin End Metab* **92**: 405–13.

Vermuelen A, Verdonck L, Kaufman JM. (1999). A critical evaluation of simple methods for estimation of free testosterone in serum. *J Clin Endocrinol Metab* **84**: 3666–72.

Zitzmann M, Faber S, Nieschlag E. (2006). Association of specific symptoms and metabolic risks with serum testosterone in older men. *J Clin Endocrinol Metab* **91**: 4335–43.

Chapter 4

Primary hypogonadism

Arif Hamda and Pierre-Marc Bouloux

> **Key points**
>
> - The majority of cases of primary hypogonadism are associated with failure of testosterone production and spermatogenesis.
> - Klinefelter's Syndrome is the commonest cause of primary hypogonadism occurring in approximately 1 in 500 male births.
> - Congential causes of hypogonadism are associated with cryptorchidism – failure of one or both testicles to descend.
> - Maldescent of the testis increases the risk of subsequent development of testicular cancer by 10%.
> - Congential causes of primary hypogonadism are associated with tall stature due to failure of epiphyseal closure and eunuchoid body shape.

4.1 Introduction

The normal testis has two functions: synthesis and secretion of androgenic hormones, particularly testosterone of Leydig cell origin, and production of mature spermatozoa in the seminiferous tubules. Although the anatomical bases of physiological control of these two processes are highly interrelated clinically in primary hypogonadism, failure of one function can occur independently of the other. In most causes of primary hypogonadism, however, there is failure in both compartments.

The malfunction of either (or both) interstitial (Leydig) cells or seminiferous tubular epithelium, in primary hypogonadism can occur either during development, or postnatally, as a consequence of acquired pathologies that damage the testes. Falls in the output of testosterone and/or the Sertoli cell product inhibin B lead, by negative feedback, to increased secretion of the gonadotrophis, luteinizing hormone (LH) and follicle-stimulating hormone (FSH), from the pituitary in an attempt to 'restore' testicular function, This leads to the typical hypergonadotrophic hypogonadism associated with primary hypogonadism. By contrast, secondary hypogonadism is due to perturbation of the hypothalamo-gonadotroph axis, resulting in failure of gonadotrophin secretion (leading to hypogonadotrophic hypogonadism).

The distinction between primary and secondary hypogonadism is made by measurement of the serum concentration of LH, FSH, and testosterone levels. Primary hypogonadism is more common than secondary hypogonadism. Although many testicular diseases damage both Leydig cells and seminiferous tubules, primary hypogonadism is more likely to be associated with a decrease in sperm production than in testosterone production. Clinical findings in hypogonadism result from either decreased spermatogenesis (causing subfertility) or decreased testosterone secretion. The latter causes a wide variety of symptoms and signs depending on the stage of life in which the deficiency occurs.

Physical signs (in male hypogonadism) include small testis size (reference range 15–25 ml, approximately 4.5 × 3.0 cm), which is seen in virtually all cases of male hypogonadism, except those of recent onset (Table 4.1). Because seminiferous tubules comprise most of the testicular volume, decline in testicular volume usually correlates directly with a decline in sperm production. Decreased testosterone production may lead to a reduction in body hair, loss of muscle mass, anaemia, arrest of temporal balding, small prostate size, and decreased libido.

Table 4.1 Effects of testosterone deficiency according to age of onset	
Age	**Clinical manifestations**
In utero	Micropenis Hypospadias Cryptorchidism Ambiguous genitalia
Peri-pubertal	Delayed or absent puberty. Eunuchoid segments Decreased phallic and testicular growth Gynaecomastia, high pitched voice Eunuchoidal body habitus Reduced peak bone mass and poor muscle development
Adulthood	Decreased libido, potency, mood and energy, subfertility and infertility Decrease in sexual hair, muscle mass, and strength Osteoporosis, anaemia Decline in cognitive skills, vitality Increased visceral fat

Gynaecomastia, which usually reflects the response to a decrease in the free androgen/oestrogen ratio, is particularly common in primary hypogonadism, where elevated LH levels stimulate aromatization of testosterone to oestradiol within the testes.

Onset of hypogonadism before epiphyseal fusion of the long bones is associated with delayed epiphyseal closure, prolonging growth of the appendicular skeleton, while retarding vertebral growth. This can therefore lead to eunuchoid proportions, in which the ratio of upper body segment (pubis to vertex) to the lower body segment (pubis to floor) is <0.9 and the arm span exceeds height by >5 cm. Primary hypogonadism may be classified as congenital or acquired.

4.2 Congenital causes

4.2.1 Klinefelter's Syndrome

This syndrome was originally described in 1942 when Klinefelter *et al.* described nine men with gynaecomastia, small testes with seminiferous tubule dysgenesis, azoospermia, and elevated gonadotrophin levels. The aneuploid basis of the disorder was subsequently established. Diagnosis requires the demonstration of one or more supernumerary X chromosomes, the 47,XXY karyotype being commonest. Klinefelter's Syndrome and its variants are the commonest cause of primary hypogonadism, occurring in approximately 1 in 500 live male births. About 90% of patients with Klinefelter's Syndrome have a non-mosaic 47,XXY (classic karyotype). The commonest mosaic form is 47,XXY/46,XY; other mosaic types are 48,XXXY, 48,XXYY and 49,XXXXY.

The 47,XXY genotype results from non-disjunction of the sex chromosomes of either parent during meiotic division in gametogenesis, while mosaicism probably results from non-disjunction during mitotic division after conception. The greater the number of extra X chromosomes, the greater the phenotypic consequences. Unlike many other aneuploidies, Klinefelter's Syndrome is not associated with an increased rate of miscarriage and most pregnancies result in live births. It is not clearly known why the extra X chromosome results in impairment of testicular function.

4.2.1.1 *Clinical features of Klinefelter's Syndrome*

Klinefelter's Syndrome is characterized by a combination of very small firm testes (1–4 ml), gynaecomastia, and hypergonadotrophic hypogonadism, which usually becomes apparent during puberty. Patients are usually inconspicuous until puberty. Men with Klinefelter's Syndrome tend to be tall (mean adult height above the 80th percentile for the population) with relatively long legs as a proportion of overall height (eunuchoid segments). At early puberty the defect in testosterone

Table 4.2 Causes of primary hypogonadism

Congenital causes:
- Klinefelter's Syndrome
- XX males
- XYY syndrome
- Noonan syndrome
- Leydig cell aplasia or hypoplasia
- Cryptorchidism
- Enzymatic defects in testosterone synthesis
- Myotonic dystrophy

Acquired causes:
- Antineoplastic and alkylating agents
- Alcohol and other medications
- Radiation
- Environmental toxins
- Orchitis
- Human immune deficiency virus (HIV)
- Testicular trauma and torsion
- Systemic diseases
- Idiopathic

secretion is often partial. In men, the diagnosis is suspected in the presence of firm testes <2 cm in length, and other clinical signs of androgen deficiency of varying degree; most patients exhibit reduced testosterone levels, reflecting increasing Leydig cells insufficiency. About half of the patients develop painless gynaecomastia shortly after the onset of puberty and mammary carcinoma is 20 times more common in Klinefelter's Syndrome. Without testosterone replacement the typical clinical signs of androgen deficiency progressively develop. The pure non-mosaic XXY patient is typically azoospermic.

Large prospective surveys show that intellectual impairment is present in many patients but the true proportion of affected individuals with subnormal intelligence is not known. Dyssocial behaviour and personality disorders are common. Difficulties in maintaining permanent employment and a tendency to ramble in conversation are recognized. Compared with other boys of their age, adolescents with Klinefelter's Syndrome consider themselves more sensitive, introspective, apprehensive, and insecure. Patients with Klinefelter's Syndrome may suffer from other conditions later in life such as chronic pulmonary diseases, germ cell tumours, diabetes mellitus, hypothyroidism, varicose veins leading to chronic leg ulcers, and taurodontism – (with early tooth decay).

4.2.1.2 *Diagnosis of Klinefelter's Syndrome*

This diagnosis is made from the clinical features and the typical hormonal profile of hypergonadotrophic hypogonadism, and is confirmed by karyotype analysis following leucocyte culture. This may demonstrate a 47,XXY or multiple cell lines in the mosaic variants. The Barr chromatin body test is a rapid test used to determine chromosomal abnormality in a swab from the buccal mucosa. Sometimes a skin fibroblast culture to identify other tissue karyotypes may be necessary to clearly define the more obscure mosaics.

4.2.2 **XX male**

A common variant of Klinefelter's Syndrome, the XX male is characterized by the combination of male external genitalia, testicular differentiation of the gonads, and a 46,XX karyotype. Approximately 75% of patients have Y chromosome material translocated on to the tip of the X chromosome. Translocation of a DNA segment that contains the testis determining gene (SRY: Sex Determining Region Y) from Y to the X chromosome occurs during paternal meiosis. The XX male syndrome has an incidence of 1:20,000. Most SRY-positive patients have a clinical picture very similar to Klinefelter's Syndrome (small firm testes, azoospermia, and gynaecomastia) SRY-negative XX men are less virilized than SRY-positive men and tend to have a higher incidence of genital organ malformations, such as hypospadias and maldescended testes. Karyotyping is the only way to differentiate the XX male from classical Klinefelter's Syndrome.

4.2.3 **XYY syndrome**

Most 47,XYY males have no health problems distinct from those of 46,XY males. The diagnosis depends entirely on demonstration of an extra Y chromosome, the diagnosis often being made by chance. Men with the 47,XYY syndrome have normal testicular volume, and normal testosterone and gonadotrophin levels, such that the majority of patients are well androgenized and fertile. Onset of puberty may be delayed and some patients may need testosterone replacement. Cognitive abilities may be impaired, but in contrast to previous ideas there is no evidence that men with the 47,XYY syndrome are more aggressive.

4.2.4 **Noonan syndrome**

Phenotypic and genotypic males with many of the physical signs of classic female Turner syndrome have been described under a variety of names, including Noonan syndrome and male Turner syndrome. The condition may occur sporadically or may be familial; inherited in an autosomal dominant fashion with variable penetrance. A webbed neck may be present together with short stature, low set ears, ptosis, shield-like chest, diminished spermatogenesis, cryptorchidism decreased Leydig cell function, cubitus valgus, and pulmonary stenosis. Most patients have small testes with mild to moderate hypogonadism, and the majority are infertile. Testosterone is often low, with raised gonadotrophins, which is indicative of primary hypogonadism.

4.2.5 **Myotonic dystrophy**

Myotonic dystrophy is a clinically and genetically heterogeneous disorder, characterized by cataracts, baldness, muscle weakness, and hypogonadism in 80% of affected males. It is transmitted in an autosomal dominant fashion, with marked variability in penetrance. The underlying lesion is an expansion CTG repeat in the 3´ untranslated region of a gene that encodes a serine–threonine protein kinase located on chromosome 19. Testicular histology varies from moderate derangement of spermatogenesis with germinal cell arrest to regional hyalinization and fibrosis of the seminiferous tubules. If testicular hyalinization and fibrosis are extensive then Leydig cell function may be impaired. FSH concentration is uniformly increased.

There are two types of myotonic dystrophy. About 80% of affected males with myotonic dystrophy type 1 have some degree of primary testicular failure. Oligospermia or azoospermia with infertility are common problems and serum testosterone may be slightly decreased.

Type 2 is generally a less severe disease. Testicular atrophy is not noted until adulthood, and most patients develop and maintain normal facial and body hair growth and libido.

4.2.6 **Leydig cell aplasia or hypoplasia**

This is a very rare cause of male pseudohermaphroditism with ambiguous genitalia. The condition is caused by inactivating mutations in the LH receptor that alters receptor signal transduction. Testes are often present in the inguinal canal. Patients with this condition often present in infancy with a variable degree of genital ambiguity. Mild defects may present with micropenis hypospadias and infertility.

4.2.7 **Enzyme defects of testosterone biosynthesis**

Defects of testosterone biosynthesis are very rare and due to inherited autosomal-recessive defects of genes encoding enzymes essential for testosterone synthesis (Table 4.3). These mutations usually involve the cholesterol side chain cleavage enzyme 17α-hydroxylase (17,20-lyase), or 3β-hydroxysteroid dehydrogenase. Both of these enzymes are present in the adrenal glands and the testes and as a result symptoms of hypogonadism and adrenal insufficiency can occur simultaneously. 17β-hydroxysteroid dehydrogenase is present in testes only. The external genitalia are feminized to a varying degree as these mutations result in decreased testosterone secretion in the first trimester of pregnancy.

Table 4.3 Enzymatic defects leading to hypergonadotrophic hypogonadism
• 17α-hydroxylase/17, 20-lyase deficiency
• 17-ketosteroid reductase
• 5α-reductase deficiency

4.3 Cryptorchidism (undescended testes)

Cryptorchidism by definition indicates a hidden testis. Testes normally enter the scrotum by the seventh month of intrauterine life. The pathogenesis of cryptorchidism is not well understood. The passage of testes through the inguinal canal is believed to result from interaction between mechanical and hormonal factors. The undescended testes may remain in the abdominal cavity or may be palpable in the inguinal canal or just outside the external ring. Cryptorchidism can affect one or both testes. About 10% of cases are bilateral. About 2–3% of all full-term boys have undescended testes. In two-thirds the testicle descends eventually, so that the incidence of post-pubertal cryptorchidism is <0.5%.

Malpositioning of testes increases the risk of developing testicular carcinoma by 10-fold, although surgical correction of malposition may not eliminate the risk of neoplasia. The clinical consequences depend partly on whether one or both testes are undescended. If only one testis is undescended, there is a 25% likelihood of a subnormal sperm count and the serum FSH level is slightly high. If both testes are undescended, the sperm count is generally severely impaired and the patient infertile; serum testosterone concentration may be subnormal and the patient undervirilized. Diagnosis is made by careful clinical examination. Ultrasound examination, and CT/MRI may be required to identify clinically non-palpable testes. An hCG test should be performed if neither testis is visible, to distinguish between cryptorchidism and anorchidism.

4.4 Acquired causes

4.4.1 Orchitis

Orchitis is a rare cause of hypogonadism, and the mumps orchitis infection is most closely associated with testicular damage. Testicular failure from mumps orchitis is a much more common manifestation when mumps occurs in adulthood than in childhood. The incidence of mumps orchitis is decreasing because of the widespread use of the mumps vaccine. The seminiferous tubules are almost always severely affected, often resulting in infertility, especially if both testes are involved. Leydig cells also may be affected, resulting in decreased testosterone levels. Orchitis may complicate infections with other viruses such as echovirus, lymphocytic choriomeningitis virus, varicella, coxsackie A, and group B arbovirus. Uncommon causes of orchitis include gonorrhoea, syphilis, leprosy, tuberculosis, and brucellosis.

4.4.2 **Antineoplastic and alkylating agents**

Antineoplastic drugs particularly alkylating agents are gonadotoxic. Alkylating agents such as cyclophosphamide, busulfan, melphalan, and chlorambucil can damage the seminiferous tubules to a degree leading to azoospermia and a significantly raised serum FSH level. The degree of damage is proportionate to the extent and duration and type of agent used for treatment. For example, nearly 100% of patients receiving MOPP (mechlorethamine, vincristine, procarbazine, and prednisolone) chemotherapy become azoospermic. Unlike the germinal epithelium, Leydig cells are largely resistant to antineoplastic agents and testosterone secretion is impaired to a lesser extent. Antimetabolites such as methotrexate and 5-fluorouracil impair spermatogenesis to a lesser extent. Cisplatin can lead to a decrease in sperm count, but this usually is reversible. Many other antineoplastic agents can cause some degree of seminiferous tubular damage but usually to a lesser degree than alkylating agents.

4.4.3 **Radiation**

The germinal epithelium is extremely sensitive to radiation. Direct radiation to testes as in treatment for leukaemia and lymphoma causes damage to testes, and particularly in pre-pubertal and adult men, may be potentiated by chemotherapy. The degree of the damage is proportionate to the amount of radiation exposure. Fractionated radiation may have a more profound effect than the single-dose radiation regimens. Radiation doses as low as 15 cGy transiently reduce the pool of spermatogonial cells, and 600 cGy permanently destroys germinal elements. Permanent Leydig cell damage occurs with doses of 2000–3000 cGy when used for the treatment of testicular involvement in acute lymphoblastic leukaemia. Radioactive iodine when used in high doses as in treatment of thyroid carcinoma can lead to a reduction in sperm count. Sperm banking should be performed prior to chemoradiation therapy.

4.4.4 **Environmental toxins**

Many potential environmental toxins, heavy metals, and chemicals have been shown to affect spermatogenesis in animals. The pesticide dibromochloropropane (DBCP) has been associated with infertility in farm workers using it in the fields.

4.4.4.1 *Alcohol and other drugs*

Alcohol has direct toxic effects on the testes. Alcohol inhibits 3β-hydroxysteroid dehydrogenase, an enzyme of testosterone biosynthesis, which leads to androgen deficiency. Acute alcohol consumption in healthy males leads to a reversible decrease in testosterone level with increased LH, indicating transient primary hypogonadism. Alcohol, when consumed in excess for prolonged periods, causes decreases in testosterone level, independent of liver disease or malnutrition. Testosterone levels may be low and oestradiol levels may be high in persons using marijuana, heroin, and methadone.

Many medications that are used for a variety of clinical conditions may lead to hypogonadism. In general, drugs interfere with testicular function in one of four ways: (1) inhibition of testosterone synthesis; (2) blockage of androgen action; (3) enhancement of oestrogen levels; or (4) direct inhibition of spermatogenesis. Some drugs may have multiple effects. Suramin, an antiparasitic drug, may block testosterone biosynthesis by Leydig cells. Ketoconazole and spironolactone block the synthesis of androgen by interfering with the late steps in androgen biosynthesis. Cimetidine and spironolactone compete with androgen for binding to the androgen receptor and thus block androgen action in target cells. Glucocorticoids can lead to hypogonadism via inhibition of both pituitary LH release and by a direct effect on the testes. A number of antihypertensives can cause problems with potency and ejaculation disorders.

4.4.5 **HIV**

Histological changes in testes of AIDS patients are common, such as decreased spermatogenesis, thickened basement membrane and interstitial infiltrate are often seen in autopsy series. The presence of mycobacterium, toxoplasma, and cytomegalovirus in testicular tissue is common in patients systemically infected with this virus. Men with HIV infection may have varying degrees of hypogonadism, as shown by lower serum testosterone concentration. Serum FSH and LH can be elevated or normal indicating both primary and secondary hypogonadism. Gonadal function appears to be affected more significantly in the later stages of HIV infection. Some medications used in the treatment of HIV-related conditions may alter testicular function. Hypogonadism in HIV-infected men has been observed less commonly since the introduction of retroviral therapy.

4.4.6 **Testicular trauma and torsion**

The exposed position of testes in the scrotum renders them susceptible to both thermal and physical trauma, particularly in individuals with hazardous occupations. Testicular torsion can cause permanent damage if not treated promptly.

4.4.7 **Systemic diseases**

Many chronic and systemic diseases cause hypogonadism both by a direct testicular effect and by decreasing gonadotrophin secretion (see Table 4.4). Sickle cell disease is also associated with low testosterone levels in conjunction with raised gonadotrophins.

Table 4.4 Systemic disorders associated with hypogonadism
• Liver cirrhosis
• Chronic renal failure
• Chronic anaemia (sickle cell disease, thalassaemia major)
• Haemochromatosis
• Gastrointestinal diseases (Crohn's disease, coeliac disease)
• Thyroid diseases
• Cardiac diseases (congestive cardiac failure)
• Respiratory diseases (cystic fibrosis, chronic obstructive pulmonary disease)
• Cushing syndrome
• Diabetes mellitus
• Amyloidosis
• Granulomatous diseases

Key references

Adler RA. (1992). Clinically important effects of alcohol on endocrine function. *J Clin Endocrinol Metab* **74**: 957–60.

Alman J, Brenner PP, McDonald PC. (1980). Androgen and estrogen production in elderly men with gynecomastia and testicular atrophy after mumps orchitis. *J Clin Endocrinol Metab* **50**: 380.

Barthold JS, Gonzalez R. (2003). The epidemiology of congenital cryptorhidism, testicular ascent and orchidopexy. *J Urol* **170**: 2396.

Block RI, Farinpour R, Schlechte JA. (1992). Effects of chronic marijuana use on testosterone, luteinizing hormone, follicle-stimulating hormone, prolactin and cortisol in men and women. *Drug Alcohol Depend* **28**: 121–8.

Brauner R, Czernichow P, Cramer P et al. (1983). Leydig cell function in children after direct testicular irradiation for acute lymphoblastic leukemia. *N Engl J Med* **309**: 25.

Danesi R, La RoccaRV, Cooper MR et al. (1996). Clinical and experimental evidence of inhibition of testosterone production by suramin. *J Clin Endocrinol Metab* **81**: 2238.

De la Chapelle A, Koo GC, Wachtel SS. (1978). Recessive sex-determining genes in human XX male syndrome. *Cell* **l5**: 837–42.

Fenchner PY, Marcantonio SM, Jaswaney V, Stetten G, Goodfellow PN, Milgen CJ, Smith KD, Bdrkovitz. (1993). The role of the sex-determining region Y gene in etiology of 46, XX maleness. *J Clin Endocrinol Metab* **76**: 690–5.

Ferguson-Smith MA, Cooke A, Affara NA, Boyd E, Tolmie JE. (1990). Genotype-phenotype correlations in XX males and their bearing on current theories of sex determination. *Hum Genet* **84**: 198–202.

Friedman NM, Plymate SR. (1980). Leydig cell dysfunction and gynecomastia in adult males treated with alkylating agents. *Clin Endocrinol* **12**: 553.

Handelsman DJ, Turtle JR. (1983). Testicular damage after radioactive iodine (I-13 1) therapy for thyroid cancer. *Clin Endocrinol* **18**: 465.

Klinefelter HF Jr, Reifenstein EC Jr. (1942). Albright F. Syndrome characterized by gynecomastia, spermatogenesis, without aleydigism and increased secretion of follicle stimulating hormone. *J Clin Endocrinol Metab* **2**: 6l5–22.

Kogan S. (1987). Fertility in cyptorchidism. An overview in 1987. *Eur J Pediatr* **146 (Suppl. 2)**: S21.

Lampe H, Horwich A, Norman A *et al.* (1997). Fertility after chemotherapy for testicular germ cell cancers. *J Clin Oncol* **15**: 239.

Leonard JM, Bremner WJ, Capell PT, Paulsen CA. (1975). Male hypogonadism: Klinefelter and Reifenstein syndrome. *Birth Defects* **11**: 17–22.

Lo JC, Schambelan M. (2001). Reproductive function in human immunodeficiency virus infection. *J Clin Endocrinol Metab* **86**: 2338.

Martin DC. (1982). Malignancy in the cryptorchid testis. *Urol Clin North Am* **9**: 371.

Meola G. (2000). Clinical and genetic heterogeneity in myotonic dystrophies. *Muscle Nerve* **23**: 1789.

Netley C. (1987). Predicting intellectual functioning in 47,XXY boys from characteristics of sibs. *Clin Genet* **32**: 24–7.

Pillai SB, Besner GE. (1998). Paediatric testicular problems. *Paediatr Clin North Am* **45**: 813.

Pont A, Williams PL, Azhar S, *et al.* (1982). Ketoconazole blocks testosterone synthesis. *Arch Intern Med* **142**: 2137.

Poretsky L, Can S, Zumoff B. (1995). Testicular dysfunction in human immunodeficiency virus infected men. *Metabolism* **44**: 946.

Qureshi MS, Pennington JH, Goldsmith HJ, Cox PE. (1972). Cyclophosphamide therapy and sterility. *Lancet* **ii**: 1290.

Shapiro E, Kinsella TJ, Makuch RW, *et al.* (1985). Effects of fractionated irradiation on endocrine aspects of testicular function. *J Clin Oncol* **3**: 1232.

Theilgaard A. (1993). Aggression and the XYY personality. *Int J Law Psychiatry* **6**: 413–21.

Vazquez JA, Pinies JA, Martul P, *et al.* (1990). Hypothalmic-pituitary-testicular function in 70 patients with myotonic dystrophy. *J Endocrinol Invest* **13**: 375.

Watson AR, Rance CP, Bain J. (1985). Long-term effects of cyctophosphamide on testicular function. *Br Med J* **291**: 1475.

Whorton D, Krauss RM, Marshall S, *et al.* (1997). Fertility in male pesticide workers. *Lancet* **ii**: 1259.

Chapter 5

Secondary hypogonadism

Richard Quinton

> ### Key points
> - Secondary hypogonadism is not a final diagnosis: hypopituitarism, hyperprolactinaemia, and/or a parasellar lesion must always be considered.
> - Micropenis, scrotal hypoplasia, and/or bilateral cryptorchidism in an infant strongly suggest congenital secondary hypogonadism, and referral to a paediatric endocrinologist is necessary.
> - Pituitary tumours associated with hyperprolactinaemic hypogonadism must not be automatically assumed to be prolactinomas.
> - Secondary hypogonadism is an under-appreciated feature of both critical illness and chronic disease.
> - It is one of the very few treatable causes of male infertility.

5.1 Introduction

Secondary hypogonadism (SH) defines testicular dysfunction arising from disorders of the hypothalamus or pituitary gland resulting in deficient gonadotrophin [luteinizing hormone (LH) and follicle-stimulating hormone (FSH)] secretion. The serum testosterone level is low, accompanied by low or 'inappropriately' normal gonadotrophins, and oligospermia or azoospermia. The testes are quiescent because they are unstimulated, but retain the potential for normal secretory and spermatogenic function.

5.2 Neurohumoral regulation of the male reproductive axis

5.2.1 Developmental biology of the gonadotrophin-releasing hormone pulse generator

Certain developmental preconditions are required for the establishment of a fully functioning hypothalmo-pituitary–testicular axis (Figure 2.3).

- Migration of gonadotrophin-releasing hormone (GnRH)-secreting neurons from their extracranial site of origin in the embryonic olfactory placode to their 'adult' location distributed throughout the mediobasal hypothalamus.
- These 1–2000 neurons mature into a neural network delivering episodic, synchronized secretory bursts, modulated by inputs from sex steroids and multiple neurotransmitters/neuropeptides: the GnRH pulse generator.
- Pulsatile release of GnRH into the hypophyseoportal circulation stimulates release of LH and FSH from anterior pituitary gonadotroph cells (whereas continuous infusion of GnRH or treatment with a long-acting GnRH analogue instead downregulates gonadotrophin secretion, thereby inducing a state of iatrogenic SH).

5.3 Baseline evaluation of men with secondary hypogonadism

A detailed list of the causes of SH is given in Table 5.1 and a comprehensive list of investigations in Table 5.2, but the following questions are central to the initial evaluation:

- Does the 9 a.m. serum biochemistry indicate severe SH (serum LH and FSH <2.0 U/l; total testosterone <6 nmol/l) or more borderline hypogonadism (LH and FSH 2–6 U/l; total testosterone 6–11 nmol/l)?
- Does the history suggest a congenital disorder (e.g. cryptorchidism ± micropenis, failure to initiate/progress through puberty) or has hypogonadism developed in later life?
- Is there broader hypopituitarism or isolated SH?
- Are there non-reproductive phenotypic abnormalities, such as anosmia or short stature? (Tables 5.1 and 5.2).
- Are there features of a parasellar lesion, such as headache or visual field defect.
- Is the patient systemically unwell or carrying a significant disease burden?
- Do blood tests raise the possibility of iron overload or coeliac disease?

Pituitary MRI is indicated for men with:

- Severe SH in the absence of obvious critical illness or chronic disease process
- SH and evidence of broader hypopituitarism.
- SH and suspected parasellar mass effect
- SH and elevated serum PRL.

5.4 **Isolated hypogonadotrophic hypogonadism (IHH)**

5.4.1 **Aetiology, prevalence, and developmental basis of isolated hypogonadotrophic hypogonadism**

IHH is defined by hypothalamic deficiency of GnRH or, more rarely, pituitary resistance to GnRH action, resulting in biochemically severe SH. The defect is congenital and presumed to be entirely genetically based. Pituitary MRI is normal and causes of functional or organic gonadotrophin suppression cannot be identified (Table 5.1).

Table 5.1		
1. Congenitally programmed		
(a) Isolated hypogonadotrophic hypogonadism (IHH)		
Kallmann's Syndrome: IHH +anosmia	*KAL1, NELF*	*FGFR1, FGF8,*
normosmic IHH	*GnRHR, GPR54*	*PRK2, PRKR2*
adult-onset normosmic IHH	*FGF8, PKR2*	
IHH ± anosmia with reversal	*GnRHR, FGFR1, KAL PKR2*	
(b) Other congenital syndromes associated with SH		
Adrenohypoplasia congenita (AHC)	*DAX1*	
SH + childhood-onset morbid obesity	*Leptin, LeptinR, PC1*	
SH + mental retardation + obesity Prader-Willi Bardet–Biedl	deletions within paternally imprinted 15q11.2–12. region *BBS1–11* (multiple chromosomal loci)	
CHARGE syndrome	*CHD7* mutations found in 2/3 of cases	
(c) Combined pituitary hormone deficiency (CPHD)		
No extrapituitary phenotype	*PROP1*—by far the most common genetic cause of CPHD (50% of familial probands, but only 1% of sporadic cases)	
Short, rigid cervical spine	*LHX3*	
Septo-optic dysplasia (SOD), agenesis of corpus callosum	*HESX1* (mutations in <1%) a non-genetic *in utero* vascular or teratogenic insult may be responsible for most cases	
X-linked mental retardation + hypopituitarism	*SOX3* (either inactivating mutations or gene duplications)	
Anophthalmia/microphthalmia, learning difficulties, sensorineural hearing loss, oesophageal atresia, abnormal corpus callosum	*SOX2*	

Table 5.1 (*Contd.*)
2. Acquired
(a) Functional hypogonadism: gonadotrophin secretion suppressed by illness
Hyperprolactinaemia
Hypoleptinaemia, typically from eating disorder
Critical illness
Chronic systemic illness (including obesity and diabetes)
Use/abuse of androgens, progestogens, and anabolic steroids
GnRH analogue therapy
Chronic glucocorticoid treatment
Chronic opiate administration
(b) Organic disease of the parasellar region causing gonadotroph damage or unresponsiveness
Benign tumours: local pressure effect and/or treatment by surgery and/or external beam radiotherapy, e.g. pituitary adenomas, craniopharyngiomas, Rathkes's cleft cysts, and parasellar meningiomas.
Trauma: skull base trauma was always recognized to have the potential for severing the pituitary stalk, but hypopituitarism, including SH, is becoming increasingly recognized following head injuries in general.
Pituitary iron overload: especially hereditary haemochromatosis.
Infiltrative diseases, e.g. neurosarcoidosis, Langerhan's cell histiocytosis, Wegener's granulomatosis, lymphocytic hypophysitis.
Post-CNS infection, especially tuberculous meningitis in the developing world.
Idiopathic – though an hitherto occult illness may yet declare itself with time.

The male prevalence is about 0.025% and affected males outnumber females some three- to fivefold. About 50% of cases have congenital anosmia and this association defines Kallmann's Syndrome. The unifying explanation for X-linked Kallmann's Syndrome rests with the description of a single 19-week human fetus carrying an Xpter chromosomal deletion, in which neuronal disconnectivity between nose and forebrain left the entire GnRH neuron populations marooned extracranially (Figure 5.1).

5.4.2 Clinical features of isolated hypogonadotrophic hypogonadism

Fifteen per cent of patients are presumptively diagnosed in childhood and 75% are diagnosed when they present with absent or arrested-early puberty. Smaller numbers present with primary infertility, osteoporosis or myopathy, or via family studies of affected probands. Fifty per cent of IHH men give a history of childhood cryptorchidism (bilateral in 70% of cases) and/or micropenis; therfore, this confirms the need for robust urological and paediatric surgical guidelines mandating paediatric endocrine assessment of boys with testicular maldescent.

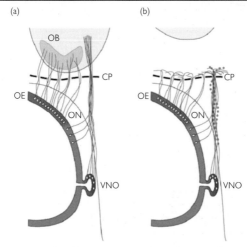

Figure 5.1 Appearance of normal, compared with KAL1-deleted, human fetus at 19 weeks gestation

(a)

(b)

Axon fascicles arising from olfactory sensory neurons (ON) in the olfactory epithelium (OE) and from (putative pheromonal chemosensory) neurons of vomeronasal organ (VNO) project through the cribriform plate (CP) to synapse within the overlying olfactory bulbs (OB). GnRH neurons have already completed their migration to the hypothalamus.

Abnormal development pattern in a 19-week fetus with X-linked Kallmann's Syndrome. The olfactory bulbs are dysplastic, the olfactory nerves have failed to make synaptic contact with the forebrain and GnRH neurons are marooned extracranially within the nasal septum and cribriform plate region.

Both IHH and constitutionally delayed puberty are three to five times more prevalent in males than females being able to distinguish between them precisely may not be possible at the initial consultation. However, features pointing towards IHH include:

- older age of patient
- tall stature
- history of cryptorchidism and/or micropenis
- presence (or history) of IHH-associated non-reproductive phenotype (Table 5.2)
- family history of IHH
- growth spurt and development of secondary sexual characteristics induced by testosterone therapy, but without concomitant testicular enlargement.

Table 5.2 Most common non-reproductive phenotypes associated with isolated hypogonadotrophic hypogonadism

- Anosmia (~50%)
- Sensorineural deafness (6–10%)
- Craniofacial defects, especially clefting (suggests *FGFR1* defect)
- Mirror movements (seen in 60–80% of Kallmann's Syndrome cases mediated by *KAL1*; <10% of *FGFR1*)
- Unilateral renal aplasia (seen in 25–30% of Kallmann's Syndrome cases mediated by *KAL1*)

5.4.3 Genetics of isolated hypogonadotrophic hypogonadism

Although most cases occur sporadically, three modes of inheritance have long been apparent (Table 5.1): X-linked recessive (e.g. KAL1), autosomal dominant with variable penetrance ± facial clefting (e.g. FGFR1, PRK2, PRK2R), and autosomal recessive (e.g. GnRHR, GPR54). The most severe endocrine phenotype is caused by KAL1 mutations, where there is near 100% anosmia, complete LH apulsatility, up to 80% prevalence of cryptorchidism, 60–80% of mirror movements, and 20–30% of renal aplasia. By contrast the 'FGFR1 phenotype' encompasses normosmia with reproductive normality, normosmic IHH, isolated anosmia, through to complete Kallmann's Syndrome.

Digenic Kallmann's Syndrome has recently been described in a male heterozygous for inherited mutations of both FGFR1 and NELF and other oligogenic cases have since been identified, indicating the presence of IHH allelic mutants within the general population. Even though rapid progress is presently being made in this field, the genetic basis for over 70% of cases remains unknown. None of the genes presently known contributes to more than 10% of the total cases and, in fact, most contribute well under 5%.

5.4.4 Newly recognized isolated hypogonadotrophic hypogonadism phenotypes

IHH was considered to be a lifelong condition, with affected men unable to complete puberty without replacement therapy. However, a small subset present with idiopathic adult-onset SH, having previously exhibited a normal puberty and reproductive phenotype. These men may also harbour mutations of IHH genes (Table 5.1).

Even more remarkable, up to 10% of men presenting with apparently classical IHH, including Kallmann's Syndrome, will eventually undergo complete 'awakening' of endogenous gonadotrophin-driven testosterone secretion, which enables them to discontinue androgen replacement therapy. This syndrome of 'IHH-with-Reversal' is distinct from simple pubertal delay because of the more advanced age of initial presentation (typically mid-20s) and of subsequent reversal (typically mid-30s), and because they may also harbour mutations of IHH genes (Table 5.1).

5.5 Combined pituitary hormone deficiency (CPHD)

The mode of presentation is highly variable, depending upon the tempo and extent of hypopituitarism. The most severely affected cases present with neonatal panhypopituitarism (hypoglycaemia, hypotension, jaundice, and failure to thrive) and non-pituitary defects. However, milder forms of CPHD are increasingly recognized, in which there is progressive, stepwise onset of pituitary dysfunction during childhood or even adult life.

We have observed the typical MRI appearances of CPHD (shallow, hypoplastic sella and ectopic posterior pituitary bright spot) in a middle-aged man presenting with SH who had previously undergone normal growth and puberty, attained full adult stature, and fathered children. Further evaluation revealed coexisting growth hormone (GH) deficiency and over time he progressed to partial thyrotroph insufficiency (see Figure 5.2).

Table 5.1 lists the gene defects presently known to cause SH as part of CPHD; all of these resulted in impaired expression of transcription factors necessary for differentiation of embryonic pituitary cell lineages. Nevertheless, the overwhelming majority of cases occur sporadically and may result from vascular or teratogenetic insults during embryonic development rather than being genetically based. There is a strong, albeit unproven suggestion that the escalating incidence of septo-optic dysplasia in the offspring of young mothers may stem from maternal substance abuse.

5.6 Organic diseases of the hypothalamus and pituitary

5.6.1 Structural lesions of the hypothalamus and pituitary gland

About three-quarters of clinical cases of hypopituitarism result from pituitary adenomas and/or their treatment. These are conventionally divided into microadenomas (<1 cm) and macroadenomas (>1 cm), with only 10% of microadenomas having the potential to grow into macroadenomas. Because of the stereotypic way that pituitary dysfunction develops in response to any kind of insult, LH and FSH (along with GH) are typically the first hormones to be 'lost'.

Parasellar tumours of extrapituitary origin (e.g. craniopharyngiomas, Rathke's cleft cysts, and meningiomas) comprise a further 15% of cases, with the balance made up of rare disorders, including lymphocytic hypophysitis, neurosarcoid, Langerhan's cell histiocytosis, pituitary

Figure 5.2 Sagittal T1-weighted MRI showing typical appearance of CPHD

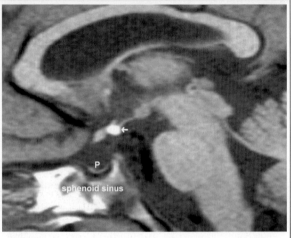

The pituitary fossa (P) is hypoplastic and the posterior pituitary bright spot is ectopic (arrowed). Resolution 1.5 Tesla.

abscess, metastasis, and Sheehan syndrome. Diagnostic accuracy is enhanced by dedicated pituitary MRI protocols, with image interpretation by a specialist neuroradiologist.

Hormone replacement and interval monitoring of tumour size may be the most appropriate course of action for a non-secretory tumour causing no mass effect, particularly in the frail and elderly. Transsphenoidal selective adenomectomy (TSA) is almost invariably deployed for adenomas secreting adrenocorticotrophic hormone or GH or causing mass effect. A transcranial approach is generally undertaken for other parasellar tumours.

Radiotherapy is increasingly reserved for tumour regrowth after initial debulking as an alternative to repeat TSA. Although modern, multiportal fractionated external beam radiotherapy regimens are probably less prone to cause hypopituitarism, annual endocrine evaluation for at least 10 years afterwards is still prudent.

Figure 5.3 Coronal T1-weighted contrast MRI showing prolactinoma at presentation

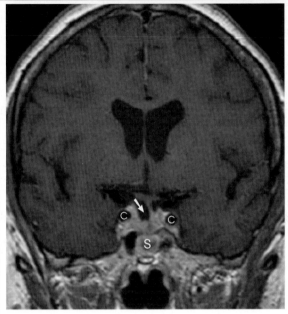

There is extension bilaterally into the cavernous sinuses (C = internal carotid arteries) and inferiorly into the sphenoid sinus (S). The pituitary stalk deviates to the left and the pituitary fossa is enlarged, but is partially empty of tissue on the right (small arrow) consistent with partial tumour infarction and, indeed, the patient gave a history of sudden-onset incapacitating headache 7 years previously. Resolution 1.5 Tesla.

Previously unsuspected pituitary macroadenomas may spontaneously undergo haemorrhagic infarction (pituitary apoplexy). Figure 5.3 illustrates the MR appearance of a man presenting with SH and serum PRL levels of 7000 U/l. Tumour has invaded the sphenoid and cavernous sinuses and the pituitary stalk; though the bony sella is enlarged it is largely empty of tissue. The patient recalled having been incapacitated with a severe headache 7 years previously, when the intrasellar tumour component probably auto-infarcted.

5.6.2 **Disorders of pituitary hormone hypersecretion**

With the exception of hyperprolactinaemia resulting from drugs, stress, or pituitary stalk compression or transection, secretory pituitary adenomas are invariably responsible for hormone excess syndromes.

Because of the local or systemic inhibitory action of the abnormally secreted hormone on gonadotrophin secretion, even a microadenoma secreting PRL, GH, or adrenocorticotrophic hormone can cause profound SH. Supraphysiological levels of PRL and, to a lesser extent, GH directly suppress gonadotrophin secretion, as does adrenocorticotrophic hormone-stimulated hypercortisolaemia. In both acromegaly and pituitary Cushing's disease, suppression of gonadotrophin secretion also arises from chronic disease burden (which may include diabetes or sleep apnoea syndrome).

5.7 **Hyperprolactinaemia**

5.7.1 **Lactotroph adenomas**

Prolactinomas account for 30–40% of clinically recognized pituitary adenomas. In the absence of a menstrual cycle, men (and/or their physicians) may not recognize the progressive onset of hypogonadism, resulting in delayed diagnosis. Thus, although the apparent prevalence in males is lower, mean tumour size at presentation is significantly greater than in women. Although TSA remains an option for selected cases most patients tolerate dopamine agonists well, with normalization of serum PRL and tumour shrinkage, often with resolution of SH. Serum PRL is indicative of prolactinoma size and biochemical surveillance (rather than routine MRI) can thus suffice thereafter; hence the vital importance of making an accurate diagnosis.

5.7.2 **Diagnostic pitfalls**

Tumour mass effect can disrupt pituitary stalk function, thereby releasing normal pituitary lactotrophs from tonic dopaminergic inhibition; therefore even a non-secreting tumour can cause serum PRL elevation. Obviously, the smaller the tumour and the higher the PRL level, the greater the pre-test probability of prolactinoma and a wide range of serum PRL cut-offs has been proposed. However, the safest course is to defer making a definitive diagnosis of prolactinoma until the tumour has unequivocally reduced in size from one MRI scan to the next while being treated with dopamine agonists.

5.7.3 **Causes of hyperprolactinaemia**

Apart from pituitary adenomas, elevated prolactin levels are found in association with renal failure, primary hypothyroidism, liver cirrhosis, and drug treatment (commonly includes sulpiride, haloperidol, risperidone, tricyclic antidepressants, domperidone, and metoclopramide – see below). If after investigation a cause is not identified and there is significant and persistent elevation of the serum prolactin level then this is known as idiopathic or non-tumour hyperprolactinaemia.

5.8 Functional suppression of gonadotrophin secretion

5.8.1 Critical illness

Critical illness of any kind can cause severe SH, with the biochemical degree of hypogonadism being directly related to the severity of illness. The mechanism is multifactorial, but probably includes enhanced aromatization of androgens to oestrogens, circulating inflammatory cytokines (especially interleukin 6), hypercortisolaemia (or administered glucocorticoids), hyperprolactinaemia (from stress or antidopaminergic drugs), and, potentially, opioid analgesia. There are no data on whether SH in this context is an adaptive or maladaptive physiological response, i.e. helpful or harmful to recovery from critical illness.

Given that thyroid hormone biochemistry can also be abnormal as part of a non-thyroidal illness syndrome, distinguishing critical illness from hypopituitarism is not always straightforward (particularly following head injury). However, an elevated serum cortisol (retrospectively assayed if necessary from the admission blood sample) points away from organic hypopituitarism.

5.8.2 Chronic systemic illness

Although similar mechanisms are involved, hypogonadism is generally less severe than in critical illness. Obesity, type 2 diabetes, cardiovascular disease, AIDS, cirrhosis, and chronic renal failure have all been shown to be associated (Table 5.1). Finally, it is always worth screening patients for occult coeliac disease or haemochromatosis.

5.8.3 Prescribed medication and drugs of abuse

Mild degrees of hyperprolactinaemic SH are ubiquitous among men being treated for major psychiatric disease with conventional antidopaminergic agents, particularly sulpiride or risperidone. When the resulting hypogonadism is more severe the optimal solution is for the patient's psychiatrist to switch to a drug such as clozapine, quetiapine, olanzapine, or lithium. Normalization of serum PRL level with resolution of SH indicates that no further investigation is required. When it is not feasible to make radical amendments to neuroleptic medication, pituitary MRI is required to exclude a mass lesion and judicious androgen replacement should be considered, particularly if bone density is impaired. Although verapamil and virtually all the anti-emetics can also elevate serum PRL, it is unusual for these to result in significant SH.

The suppressive effect of sex steroids on gonadotrophin secretion can last for many months after discontinuation, during which time SH persists; this constitutes a potent disincentive for athletes or body builders to abstain long enough for their reproductive axes to recover. 'Underground' websites advocate aromatase inhibitors or selective oestrogen receptor modulators in an attempt to prevent (or shorten) the duration of SH in androgen abusers; however, hard evidence of efficacy is lacking despite a reasonable theoretical basis. Combined therapy with androgens and progestagens is so effective at suppressing gonadotrophin secretion and spermatogenesis that phase III trials of various regimens are presently being undertaken for male contraception.

Chronic treatment with either opiates (for pain or dependence) or glucocorticoids for inflammatory disease can also lead to SH, although the effect is hard to disentangle from that of the underlying chronic disease process.

Key references

Gillam MP, Molitch ME, Lombardi G, Colao A. (2006). Advances in the treatment of prolactinomas. *Endocr Rev* **27**: 485–534.

Kelberman D, Dattani MT. (2007). Hypothalamic and pituitary development: novel insights into the aetiology. *Eur J Endocrinol* **157**: S3–14.

Layman LC. (2007). Hypogonadotropic hypogonadism. *Endocrinol Metab Clin North Am* **36**: 283–96.

Mutch DM, Clément K. (2006). Unravelling the genetics of human obesity. *PLoS Genet* **2(12)**: e188.

Spratt DI, Cox P, Orav J, Moloney J, Bigos T. (1993). Reproductive axis suppression in acute illness is related to disease severity. *J Clin Endocrinol Metab* **76**: 1548–54.

Chapter 6

Late-onset hypogonadism

Michael Zitzmann

> ### Key points
>
> - Late-onset hypogonadism (LOH) is a frequent, but not omnipresent or mandatory clinical entity in men.
> - Classical symptoms of hypogonadism are often blurred by co-morbidities in older men.
> - Older men with LOH may benefit from testosterone substitution, mentally as well as physically, as well-being, metabolism, bone density, erythropoiesis, and body composition improve.
> - Transdermal testosterone preparations should be preferred for the substitution of testosterone in patients with LOH.
> - Safety and surveillance of this therapy are especially required with regard to the prostate and haematocrit.

I heard the old, old men say,
'Everything alters,
And one by one we drop away.'
They had hands like claws, and their knees
Were twisted like the old thorn-trees
By the waters.
I heard the old, old men say,
'All that's beautiful drifts away
Like the waters.'

William Butler Yeats

Do not go gentle into that good night,
Old age should burn and rave at close of day;
Rage, rage against the dying of the light.

Dylan Thomas

These two poems nicely show the contrast of symptoms related to age and the wish (and possibility?) to maintain vigour and strength. A translation of these metaphorical lines into physiology and modern medicine exists in the clinical entity of late-onset hypogonadism.

6.1 **Introduction**

Senescence in men as such does not imply the necessity for testosterone substitution, whereas male hypogonadism is a prerequisite for testosterone substitution. As the incidence of hypogonadism increases with age, the terms 'andropause', 'PADAM' ('partial androgen deficiency in ageing men') or 'male climacteric' have emerged in several publications, alluding to the female menopause and indicating that in men there could be an end to gonadal steroid production and fertility, which occurs as precipitously and as definitely as in women. However, a drastic decrease in androgen production cannot be observed in healthy men; androgen depletion is a rather slow process and 'andropause' turns out to be a misnomer.

Unlike the impressive somatic character of symptoms encountered with diseases associated with 'classical hypogonadism' (e.g. Kallmann's Syndrome, pituitary insufficiency, Klinefelter's Syndrome) or conditions that occur after bilateral orchidectomy, complaints of older men may be attributed to 'normal ageing processes' or illnesses associated with advancing age (e.g. diabetes mellitus or atherosclerosis). The effects of these disease entities on libido, reactive erectile function and nocturnal erections are well known, but the effects of low testosterone levels may also be an additional adverse factor. Furthermore, androgens have psychotropic effects so that a deficiency may result in depressed mood, and general fatigue, decrease in cognitive functions and intellectual activity. Older men in a hypogonadal state may also present with anaemia, as testosterone acts positively on erythropoiesis. Hypogonadism represents a risk factor for the loss of bone mass, and, can thus cause osteoporotic fractures in men. Androgen depletion can also cause loss of muscle mass and increasing body fat content. A major sign of hypogonadism in younger men is a small prostate, which is rather unlikely in older males.

Testosterone levels show great inter individual variability with advancing age; nevertheless, the proportion of men presenting with testosterone levels in the subnormal range (below 12 nmol/l) increases significantly. Longitudinal studies, such as those in populations of ageing men from Baltimore or Massachusetts, demonstrate that such low levels can be found in fewer than 1% of men aged below 40 years, but in more than 20% of men older than 60 years, and over 40% in men above 80 years.

Hence, subnormal testosterone levels are not a general but are a frequent feature of ageing men. This age-related deterioration of androgen production can be seen as a combined dysfunction of both the central and peripheral parts of the sex steroid regulation system, and is named 'late-onset hypogonadism' (LOH). The direction as well as the weighting of pathological processes within such an imbalance may vary, and LOH presents with low to low-normal testosterone concentrations and LH levels, which may be slightly decreased, normal, or elevated. In fact, the clinical entity might as well be named 'mixed hypogonadism' as there is no clear-cut definition of age in relation to LOH. Usually described as a disease of 'ageing' men, the nosology with its typical hormone constellations can also be found in men of a 'younger age'. In principle, the diagnosis of LOH is made after excluding all other causes of hypogonadism.

A central clinical question is whether the decrease of androgen levels described as LOH translates physiologically. Such clinical evidence could be sought in similarities between the symptoms of men with LOH and of other hypogonadal men, as well as the general symptoms of ageing men. In this regard, one has to be aware that ageing is most often accompanied by a decline in many physiological, cognitive, and sexual functions, as the incidence and prevalence of chronic diseases affecting these parameters increases with ageing. Such chronic diseases are mainly atherosclerosis, diabetes mellitus, and obesity. Thus, in view of the multifactorial origin of ageing symptoms, the effects of LOH may not be easy to detect. However, evidence from hypogonadism in younger men suggests a range of androgen-dependent functions, for which adverse affects caused by LOH can be assumed. In particular, the beneficial effects of testosterone substitution on these morbidities provide evidence for a significant role for androgens within the symptomatology of elderly men with LOH. These will be discussed in the following sections.

6.2 **General diagnostic approaches to male hypogonadism**

A diagnosis of LOH is made by excluding other morbidities resulting in androgen deficiency.

Hypogonadism manifests itself with a variety of symptoms that can be psychological, cognitive, sexual, as well as somatic in nature. The time of onset plays a significant part in the pattern of clinical manifestations of hypogonadism; also significant is the actual serum concentration of testosterone, leading to a stepwise increase of symptoms with decreasing testosterone levels. Older hypogonadal men usually exhibit characteristics similar to younger patients, but possibly to a lower degree. The pattern of complaints in older men may be caused at least partly by various other chronic illnesses related to the ageing process.

Once a patient presents with symptoms suggestive of androgen deficiency, standardized patterns of diagnostics and treatment should be followed. Underlying causes of hypogonadism are determined according to where they occur; at the testicular source of testosterone;

the Leydig cells (primary hypogonadism); or at the central regulation unit, consisting of the hypothalamus and the pituitary gland (secondary hypogonadism), the latter secreting luteinizing hormone (LH), which stimulates Leydig cells.

Hypogonadal symptoms also occur in cases of target organ resistance, mostly due to inherited alterations in the androgen receptor; in this case, elevated concentrations of both testosterone and LH are found and the androgen-sensitivity index is elevated, pointing to androgen resistance (see Section 6.6).

For diagnostic purposes, in suspected male hypogonadism assessment of total testosterone, LH, follicle-stimulating hormone (FSH), prolactin, and oestradiol is helpful, as well as the calculation of free testosterone from total testosterone and sex hormone binding globulin. This complete overview of hormones classifies the clinical picture with regard to fertility and oestrogen-related features of the phenotype (e.g. fat distribution, gynaecomastia, bone density). Determination of androgen receptor genotype and concentrations of serum dihydrotestosterone should be performed in special cases of suspected androgen resistance. Questionnaires related to possible androgen deficits are not useful for screening purposes because of their low sensitivity and specificity. Nevertheless, such tools may be useful for monitoring purposes during testosterone substitution therapy.

In addition, the effects of decreasing testosterone levels are enhanced by an age-dependent increase in levels of sex-hormone binding globulin, further lowering the amount of bioavailable testosterone. It is probable that reduced levels of growth hormone and insulin-like growth factor 1, which inhibit sex-hormone binding globulin production in hepatocytes, are responsible for this phenomenon.

In cases of borderline total testosterone values and existing symptoms (see below), low concentrations of bioavailable testosterone might be taken into consideration for initiating treatment. Notwithstanding, normal limits for bioavailable testosterone have not been defined.

Generally, there is no age limit with regard to treatment with testosterone substitution. In particular, the short-acting, dose-titratable transdermal preparations provide the physician with the ability to treat men with LOH (as defined by low testosterone levels in combination with the major symptoms of hypogonadism, such as depression, loss of vigour and libido, anaemia). Testosterone levels in the low-normal to mid-normal range should be aimed for.

6.3 **Modalities of testosterone substitution**

Once the diagnosis of hypogonadism has been established, androgen replacement therapy is recommended after taking into account contraindications (e.g. prostate cancer, wish to father a child). For such a treatment, the natural hormone testosterone has to be administered to provide all physiological functions. An exception is the desired simultaneous induction of fertility in secondary hypogonadism; in this case, gonadotrophins have to be administered, as external androgens cannot induce spermatogenesis. Rather, externally administered testosterone acts as a contraceptive agent as it suppresses the secretion of gonadotrophins.

The international societies involved in drafting recommendations for the treatment of ageing men favour transdermal preparations of testosterone. Testosterone gel preparations are based on hydroalcoholic carriers and can reliably provide serum concentrations within the normal range. Resorption exhibits interindividual variability and dosing should be adapted according to effects and serum levels. This short-acting method of testosterone substitution is applied daily and is recommended for cases in which rapid responses to treatment effects might be required and to facilitate proper handling of side-effects/contraindications, especially with regard to erythropoiesis or prostate-specific antigen (PSA) levels.

6.4 Benefits of testosterone substitution

When hypogonadism is treated by testosterone substitution, symptoms caused by androgen deficiency can be expected to vanish or be ameliorated. This may require some time depending on the target organ, but the effects on mood and sexuality are usually seen within weeks.

Favourable mood changes in terms of lower rates of 'negative feelings', even amelioration of depression, as well as feeling more vigour and energy will occur with testosterone substitution. Moreover, aspects related to sexuality, such as libido, quality of sexual life, and frequency and quality of erections improve when testosterone resources are replenished. Cognitive abilities can also increase as a result of testosterone substitution.

Testosterone treatment can significantly reduce body fat content in hypogonadal men, and vice versa, it can increase lean body mass; the phenomenon is due not only to shifts in proportions, but also to absolute growth of muscle tissue. As bone tissue metabolism is positively affected by testosterone and its aromatization product oestradiol, the treatment of hypogonadal men improves bone density. The process is apparent after 6 months, but usually takes 2–3 years to reach steady state.

Hypogonadal men often present with anaemia. Irrespective of the preparation used, elevation of testosterone levels will increase haemoglobin levels in these patients. Substitution effects when using intramuscular testosterone undecanoate will reach a plateau after approximately 6–9 months. A marked variability of the haematopoietic system to respond to testosterone exists, which underlines the necessity for surveillance; in some and in particular older men, unacceptably high levels of haemoglobin and haematocrit can develop, so that the dosage has to be adjusted to prevent adverse vascular events. Such side-effects are usually seen during application of short-acting intramuscular preparations, such as testosterone enanthate.

6.4.1 Surveillance of testosterone-substituted men

The ISSAM/ISA/EAU recommendations on LOH should be considered when monitoring older men who are being treated with testosterone substitution. The prostate is an androgen-dependent organ and will generally increase in size during testosterone substitution therapy. An elevation of PSA concentrations is usually seen upon initiation of treatment. As prostate cancer and benign prostate hyperplasia have a high incidence in men, careful screening by measurement of PSA, accompanied by digital rectal exams and, if possible, transrectal ultrasound (TRUS) are recommended at fixed intervals. Pathological findings and/or PSA levels higher than 4 ng/ml should lead to (temporary) testosterone withdrawal and consultation by a specialized urologist, as well as possible prostate biopsy. In addition, changes of PSA levels over time, i.e. PSA velocity, are a useful tool to assess testosterone effects on the prostate.

To date, there is no convincing evidence that TRUS is superior to palpation. Therefore, it may be at the physician's discretion to conduct TRUS twice yearly in younger patients. Furthermore, there is no absolute need to monitor bone mineral density, if there is no evidence of osteoporosis at the start of treatment. However, as hypogonadism represents a condition leading to osteoporosis, physicians will most probably want to know the initial condition of the patient in this regard.

Monitoring of testosterone treatment in age-related decline of testosterone versus monitoring in younger patients with hypogonadism may, hence, be different. It requires clinical experience to counsel patients on an individual basis with regard to surveillance and therapy modalities.

Haematocrit will increase during testosterone substitution in hypogonadal men (see above). It should not exceed 50–52% as the risk for ischaemic events is increased beyond that threshold and should be checked regularly. Testosterone preparations avoiding high peak levels are usually safer in this regard.

Testosterone affects lipid metabolism, and substitution therapy is capable of inducing shifts in lipoprotein subfractions. These changes can be of a mixed nature and the relation to cardiovascular risk remains unclear. Lipid profiles should be assessed on a regular basis and possibly regulated by additional medications. Factors exerting adverse effects on the cardiovascular system, such as cigarette smoking and arterial hypertension, should be eliminated anyway.

6.5 Perspectives and special issues

6.5.1 Osteoporosis

Osteoporosis and fractures represent a major public health problem, not only in women but also in men. It has been estimated that by the age of 50 years, men have a risk of approximately 12–15% of having an osteoporotic fracture in later life, most commonly of the vertebra, hip, or forearm. By the age of 60 years, the risk for a non-traumatic fracture rises to 25%. In the USA, about 150,000 hip fractures occur in men each year. Because of their higher peak bone mass, men present with hip, vertebral body, or forearm fractures about 10 years later than women. Hip fractures in men result in a 30% mortality rate at 1 year after fracture versus a rate of 17% in women. Hypogonadism, i.e. androgen deficiency, has been identified as an independent risk factor for such incidences. The benefits of testosterone substitution in older men, in terms of improvement of bone mass, have repeatedly been demonstrated. It is essential that the naturally occurring testosterone molecule is used in substitution therapy, since oestradiol is the aromatization product of testosterone and plays a pivotal and independent role in enhancing bone mass.

6.5.2 Anaemia

Androgens increase erythropoiesis. This is facilitated by several pathways involving enhancement of erythropoietin secretion and independently promoting differentiation of erythroid progenitor cells. Correspondingly, hypogonadal men often present with anaemia. Testosterone substitution therapy in hypogonadal men restores red blood cell mass and, hence, oxygen supply. Under certain circumstances, polycythaemia can be induced during androgen substitution, especially when supraphysiological concentrations of testosterone are reached or patients are older. Polycythaemia or elevated haematocrit represent a risk factor for cerebral ischaemia, whereas its role in relation to cardiovascular disease remains unclear. Thus, transdermal gel preparations are a more favourable treatment option for LOH.

6.5.3 Spatial cognition

Ageing is associated with deterioration of multiple aspects of cognitive performance. Studies in humans concerning the relationship between endogenous androgen levels and cognitive performance have produced evidence that, specifically, abilities of spatial cognition are positively affected by testosterone. In particular, older men with LOH exhibit lower visuospatial abilities than eugonadal controls. It has been demonstrated that testosterone substitution improves spatial cognition in hypogonadal men, which is an oestradiol-independent effect. Cerebral imaging procedures suggest areas involved in processing spatial information, such as the ventral processing stream, are activated by testosterone.

6.5.4 **Depression**

Mood disturbances and dysthymia are frequently observed in older men and can be related to testosterone concentrations, as seen in cross-sectional studies; e.g. such as the Massachusetts Male Aging Study. Correspondingly, a depressed mood is frequently observed in hypogonadal men, a situation, which is manageable by testosterone supplementation. Administration of testosterone can benefit both psychological aspects of depression (such as depressed mood, guilt, and psychological anxiety) and somatic aspects of depression (such as sleep, appetite, and libido). Mood changes in hypogonadal men improve soon after starting treatment, and this improvement is usually maintained at a plateau reached after 2 months. Overall, enhancement of positive mood aspects is more prominent than the decrease in negative mood parameters.

6.5.5 **Metabolic syndrome**

This term relates to a nosological complex increasingly observed in affluent countries and is connected to obesity and a sedentary life-style. Type 2 diabetes mellitus is an increasing pathological entity and represents an established risk factor for the development of athero-sclerotic vascular disease. Insulin resistance is the hallmark feature of type 2 diabetes and is also an important component of the metabolic syndrome, a preclinical condition including high visceral fat content, arterial hypertension, and an inflammatory status especially present in older men with testosterone deficiency. There is evidence to suggest that testosterone is an important regulator of insulin sensitiv-ity in men. Observational studies have shown that testosterone levels are low in men with diabetes, visceral obesity, coronary artery disease, and the metabolic syndrome. Short-term interventional studies support the assumption that testosterone replacement therapy in hypogonadal men induces respective clinical improvements, also concerning

inflammatory markers and cardiac status. Hypogonadism may play a role in the pathogenesis of insulin-resistant states, and androgen replacement therapy could be a potential treatment for improve-ments in glycaemic control and reduction of cardiovascular risk, particularly in diabetic men with LOH. Nevertheless, long-term studies are required to determine the potentially beneficial role of testosterone in this regard.

6.5.6 **Erectile dysfunction**

Arterial integrity is a key component for penile cavernous vasodilation, a process leading to erection and directly regulated by androgens. It has been demonstrated that erectile dysfunction is an early marker of cardiovascular events. In particular, in hypogonadal patients, the therapeutic approach with phosphodiesterase type 5 (PDE-5) inhibitors often proves unsuccessful. There is some evidence that additional testosterone treatment in men with erectile dysfunction and low androgen levels is synergistic to PDE-5 inhibitors, especially in diabetic patients.

6.6 **Pharmacogenetic implications**

Cases of androgen resistance are often characterized by features of hypogonadism in the presence of normal testosterone concentrations. Such patients often exhibit genetic alterations of the androgen receptor, leading to a dysfunctional receptor protein and reduced/ aborted testosterone action. The clinical picture may be improved by high-dose testosterone treatment, titrated to effects in androgen target organs.

Subtle modulations of the transcriptional activity induced by the androgen receptor have also been observed and frequently assigned to a polyglutamine stretch of variable length within the N-terminal domain of the receptor protein. This stretch is encoded by a variable number of CAG triplets in exon 1 of the AR gene. Longer triplet residues mitigate binding of the androgen receptor to co-activators and facilitate decreased androgenicity. An influence of the polymorphism on androgen target tissues, such as the prostate, has been demonstrated; extending these findings to pharmacogenetic considerations, a possible modulation of androgen effects during testosterone administration has to be considered. This aspect could achieve clinical significance, especially in older men, as these patients are more likely to develop unwanted androgen-related side-effects.

6.7 **Conclusions**

In summarizing the data concerning the association of LOH with clinical signs and symptoms in elderly men, it is manifest that a clinical significance exists. Nevertheless, in many instances data quality is weak, and androgen levels are only one of the many factors determining the symptomatology of elderly men. Treatment with testosterone preparations is recommended in cases of low testosterone levels associated with the above-named symptom complexes. Special recommendations for the treatment of older men are published by International Boards.

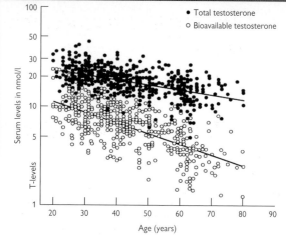

Figure 6.1 Concentration of serum testosterone in healthy men in relation to age

This study in over 500 healthy men demonstrates the relation of advancing age to lower testosterone levels. The observation is markedly stronger in bioavailable testosterone, as sex hormone binding globulin concentrations increase with advancing age (Leifke E, Gorenoi V, Wichers C, Von Zur Mühlen A, Von Büren E, Brabant G. (2000). Age-related changes of serum sex hormones, insulin-like growth factor-1 and sex-hormone binding globulin levels in men: cross-sectional data from a healthy male cohort. *Clin Endocrinol* **53**: 689–95).

Key references

Kapoor D, Goodwin E, Channer KS, Jones TH. (2006). Testosterone replacement therapy improves insulin resistance, glycaemic control, visceral adiposity and hypercholesterolaemia in hypogonadal men with type 2 diabetes. *Eur J Endocrinol* **154**: 899–906.

Kaufman JM, Vermeulen A. (2005). The decline of androgen levels in elderly men and its clinical and therapeutic implications. *Endocr Rev* **26**: 833–76.

Nieschlag E, Swerdloff R, Behre HM, Gooren LJ, Kaufman JM, Legros JJ, Lunenfeld B, Morley JE, Schulman C, Wang C, Weidner W, Wu FC. (2005). Investigation, treatment and monitoring of late-onset hypogonadism in males: ISA, ISSAM, and EAU recommendations. *Int J Androl* **28**: 125–7.

Wang C, Cunningham G, Dobs A, Iranmanesh A, Matsumoto AM, Snyder PJ, Weber T, Berman N, Hull L, Swerdloff RS. (2004). Long-term testosterone gel treatment maintains beneficial effects on sexual function and mood, lean and fat mass, and bone mineral density in hypogonadal men. *J Clin Endocrinol Metab* **89**: 2085–98.

Zitzmann M, Faber S, Nieschlag E. (2006). Association of specific symptoms and metabolic risks with serum testosterone in older men. *J Clin Endocrinol Metab* **91(11)**: 4335–43.

Chapter 7

Testosterone replacement therapy

Stefan Arver and Mikael Lehtihet

> ### Key points
>
> - Hypogonadism is a common disorder causing adverse health effects.
> - Treatment of hypogonadism is simple and straight forward.
> - Replacement doses of testosterone normalize serum levels and physiological function.
> - Treatment options include transdermal, buccal, oral, and intramuscular depot systems.
> - Side-effects of therapy are rare and risks are limited.
> - Safety monitoring include prostate and haematocrit assessment every 3 months and once yearly thereafter.

7.1 Indications

The indication for testosterone therapy in men is hypogonadism, which is a clinical syndrome complex with a combination of hypogonadal symptoms and low testosterone levels. Several new therapeutic options for testosterone replacement therapy (TRT) have become available since the mid-nineties. Although male hypogonadism with replacement to physiological concentrations is the key indication for TRT, other conditions have also been subject to testosterone therapy in the past, e.g. idiopathic male infertility, male contraception, senescence, anaemia of different origin, and delayed puberty. This chapter will only discuss TRT; use of androgens for other conditions is not covered, and the reader is referred to textbooks of internal medicine and paediatrics.

The threshold level of serum testosterone that precipitates symptoms varies for different symptoms and also between individuals. The bioactivity of testosterone will depend on the proportion of the total testosterone that is biologically active (free or bioavailable), testosterone metabolism, androgen receptor sensitivity, and post-receptor modulation. The length of the CAG repeats on the androgen receptor gene is also of clinical significance in relation to response to TRT. The normal testosterone concentration in adult men is between 8 and 35 nmol/l in fasting morning samples. Testosterone levels follow a circadian rhythm with a 20–40% difference between morning peaks and evening nadir. Samples should be drawn between 7 and 11 a.m. Samples taken after a breakfast or later in the day can cause overdiagnosis. In addition, a testosterone concentration between 10 and 12 nmol/l is a borderline value and requires additional testing, including measurement or calculation of free testosterone and/or non-sex hormone binding globulin bound testosterone (see Chapter 3).

The optimal formulation for the treatment of hypogonadism is a preparation of testosterone that normalizes the circulating testosterone level and also produces physiological levels of the two active metabolites of testosterone, oestradiol and dihydrotestosterone (DHT). The normal diurnal variation may be mimicked using a transdermal system, but the benefit of the adherence to normal physiology is unknown. Several treatment options are available with a selection of different delivery systems. The formulation can be chosen to suit the individual patient's needs for convenience without compromising treatment efficacy and safety. Natural testosterone is preferred but there are development programmes addressing different selective androgen pathways with variants of selective androgen receptor modifiers. This development has not reached clinical practice yet.

7.2 **Clinical pharmacology**

Testosterone is the key androgen. In healthy young adult men 5–10 mg of testosterone is synthesized daily with 95% derived from the testes. Testosterone interacts with a specific receptor, which is the androgen receptor genetically located in the X chromosome. Modification of testosterone is possible to enhance intrinsic androgenic potency, prolonging the duration of action, improving oral bioactivity, and increasing clinical indications. Oral intake of pure testosterone results in an extensive first hepatic pass effect, and serum levels remain unaltered even after taking gram doses of oral testosterone. Modification of the molecule by esterification with a long fatty acid enables some of the hormone to bypass the liver through lymphatic uptake; however, bioavailability is still significantly compromised.

Administration may be with transdermal, buccal, or intramuscular preparations. Despite decades of attempts to produce pharmacologically more attractive drug candidates than natural testosterone, none has so far been successful. Synthetic anabolic steroids are powerful anabolic agents but their risk of serious side-effects have made these obsolete in clinical practice.

7.3 **Testosterone replacements**

7.3.1 **Oral testosterone**

With testosterone undecanoate capsules (O-TU), an oleic acid suspension of testosterone undecanoate supposedly bypasses the liver through lymphatic uptake within the chylomicrons. O-TU has a low bioavailability and short-term action. Administration requires multiple daily dosing in conjunction with intake of fat. O-TU produces elevated levels of DHT and testosterone levels that are often below baseline levels with a paradoxical phenomenon due to the short-lived peak after each dose. Recommended doses are 120–160 mg and then 40–160 mg daily. O-TU is available in 40 mg capsules. No specific side-effects attributed to the elevated levels of DHT have been reported.

17α-alkylated testosterone derivates are still available in some countries (e.g. methyl testosterone, fluoxymesterone, stanozolol, oxandrolone, oxymetholone). The methyl group protects the molecule from liver degradation at the cost of disturbed lipoprotein metabolism (increased cholesterol) and a risk of hepatotoxicity. The 1-methyl androgen mesterolone mimics DHT, is free of hepatotoxicity but has weaker androgen effects. Both the 17α-alkylated and the 1-methyl androgen are gradually disappearing from the market.

7.3.2 **Buccal testosterone**

Testosterone can be delivered from a tablet that adheres to the buccal surface across the mucosal membrane. The tablet is convex on one side, which is placed on to the upper gum just above the lateral incisor. The tablet contains 30 mg of testosterone in a matrix with a bioadhesive polymer and is applied twice daily. Incorporation of testosterone to this matrix allows the slow release of testosterone from the tablet into the venous system, which then drains into the circulation; therefore, circumventing the hepatic first pass effect. The maximum peak circulating level is reached after 10–12 h with a C_{Max} of ~20 nmol/l. The proportion of subjects that reach the physiological testosterone range over a 24-h period is approximately 80%. The main side-effect is gum irritation. There are also difficulties with the tablets as they sometimes dislodge. Further studies would be required to fully evaluate the effect of concurrent ingestion of alcohol, tooth brushing, mouth washing, and chewing gum on the absorption of testosterone.

7.3.3 **Transdermal testosterone gels**

Hydro-alcoholic testosterone gels (1 and 2%) have become available in recent years. These gels, when applied in the morning, produce physiological serum levels almost mimicking the normal diurnal rhythm. The gel formulations contain a skin-penetration enhancer in order to enable transdermal permeation of testosterone. Ethanol is the main enhancer but there are also some systems that contain fatty acids that are known to enhance skin penetration. Testosterone gels give a bioavailability of about 10% when applied to recommended skin sites, i.e. abdomen, arms, shoulders, or thighs. The gel dries quickly and leaves marginal residues. Skin contact (direct) with women and children should be avoided for at least 2 h after application to prevent testosterone transfer. This effect is very limited once the alcohol has evaporated. Patients should avoid swimming, bathing, showering, or activities leading to excessive sweating for 2–3 h after testosterone gel administration. Product-specific side-effects are mainly application site reactions that seldom cause problems. There are currently three different preparations of testosterone gel available. The initial starting dose is 50–60 mg of testosterone per day. Physiological testosterone levels are achieved in the majority of men (Figure 7.1). Depending on serum testosterone levels dose titration may be required in some patients.

7.3.4 **Transdermal dihydrotestosterone gel**

DHT is in a hydro-alcoholic gel for dermal application and is available in some countries. The formulation is a 2.5% DHT solution that produces supraphysiological concentrations of DHT and results in normalization of the symptoms of androgen deficiency. DHT gels have been advocated for prostate safety as they disable the normal androgen accumulation mechanisms in the prostate which are based on a continuous gradient of testosterone towards the prostate by conversion of testosterone to DHT. Theoretically, a deficiency of oestrogen could occur with DHT therapy as it cannot be aromatized to form oestrogen. A recent study has provided some evidence to show that this may not be the case.

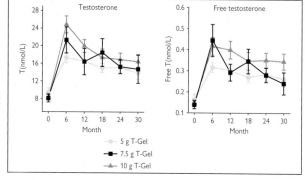

Figure 7.1 Maintenance of testosterone in the physiological range with 1% testosterone hydroalcoholic gel formulation (50 mg testosterone/5 g gel, 75 mg/7.5 g, 100 mg/10 g testosterone doses) once daily in hypogonadal men over a 30-month treatment period.

7.3.5 **Transdermal testosterone patches**

Transdermal testosterone patches have been available for both scrotal and non-scrotal applications for the last 15 years. The non-scrotal skin patches (e.g. back, upper arm, abdomen, thigh, or buttocks) ensure testosterone is continuously absorbed during the 24-h dosing period. Daily application of patches at approximately 22.00 h results in a serum testosterone concentration profile that mimics the normal circadian rhythm. Maximum concentrations occur in the early morning hours with minimum concentrations in the evening. A regimen of daily patches can maintain serum concentrations of total and free testosterone and its metabolites, DHT and 17β-oestradiol, in the mid-normal range in healthy hypogonadal men. This formula may lead to skin reactions, which are the most frequently reported adverse effects associated with testosterone patches.

Transdermal scrotal testosterone patches were the first available testosterone patches but have now been replaced by the non-scrotal patch and gels, which now dominate transdermal testosterone therapy.

7.3.6 **Intramuscular systems**

Testosterone itself has a short half-life but by esterification with fatty acids of different length the half-life after intramuscular injection can be prolonged. Esterification of position 17 with hydrophobic side chains retards hydrolysis, prolonging the half-life. The duration of the half-life is dependent on the length and structure of the side chain. The formulation is dissolved in an oil vehicle that further prolongs the absorption. A variety of esters and mixtures of esters have been used in the past, i.e. propionate, phenylpropionate isocaproate, enanthate, decanoate, and undecanoate. The longer the side chain the greater the duration of action. Testosterone undecanoate (TU) has the longest duration, thus enabling injections every 10–14 weeks.

Testosterone enanthate is a slow-acting ester with a medium long release time. Testosterone enanthate is typically injected every 2–3 weeks. Pharmacokinetics suggest that 200 mg every second week produces testosterone and metabolite levels within the reference range for the duration of the injection interval. There are major differences in serum levels prior to and the day after injection, with supraphysiological levels a few days after injection, especially levels of free testosterone. Oestradiol levels tend to be slightly above the reference range during the first half of the dosing interval. Testosterone cypionate has similar pharmacokinetics to testosterone enanthate.

TU is the most recent addition. It is a long-acting depot injection containing 1000 mg of TU dissolved in 4 ml of castor oil administered by slow intramuscular injection into the gluteal muscle. Initially two injections are given with a 6-week interval for a rapid attainment of steady-state levels (Figure 7.2). The injections are then administered

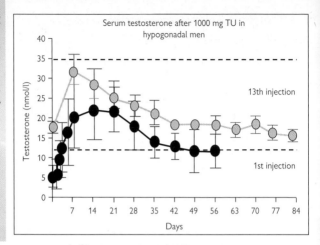

Figure 7.2 Testosterone profiles with 1000 mg testosterone undeconoate, intramuscularly, after the first and 13th injections; this demonstrates maintenance of levels within the normal physiological range.

every 10–14 weeks adjusted to maintain the trough level within the normal testosterone range. The levels of testosterone achieved generally remain within the physiological range. Its longer action and flatter testosterone concentration is preferable in many cases to testosterone enanthate. Side-effects after intramuscular administration are mainly pain or bruising at the administration site, although these are very limited.

7.3.7 **Testosterone implants**

Testosterone pellets were introduced in the 1940s and consist of pure crystalline testosterone. The implants are about the size of a wheat grain (4.5 × 12 mm) and three to six pellets of 200 mg are usually used to maintain plasma testosterone levels within the normal range for 4–6 months. Pellets have the longest duration of action of all testosterone formulations on the market. They are implanted subcutaneously with a trochar under the abdominal skin. The incision and application of the pellets will rarely lead to complications; the most common are minor bleeding, skin infection and extrusion. Pellets are available in Australia and the UK.

7.4 **Monitoring patients on testosterone replacement therapy**

Before initiation of testosterone therapy a thorough investigation is performed clarifying the indication for TRT and checking for absolute contraindications, i.e. prostate and breast cancer and relative contraindications (e.g. severe cardiac failure, severe micturition problems, elevated haematocrit, and untreated sleep apnoea). It is mandatory that prostate cancer is excluded by digital rectal examination, PSA assessment, and prostatic biopsies if indicated. Digital rectal examination and PSA should be monitored 3-monthly for the first year and annually thereafter in men over the age of 45 years. Haematocrit is checked with the same frequency, and elevation is a physiological response to TRT, though some men respond with more marked elevation than others. If that is the case several actions need to be taken: (1) check for other reasons for haematocrit elevation (sleep apnoea, chronic obstructive pulmonary disease, primary polycythaemia); (2) start low-dose aspirin therapy; (3) reduce the testosterone dose or change the regimen; (4) consider venesection. Intramuscular and implant treatment are more likely to cause elevation of the haematocrit as the testosterone levels achieved are usually higher (Dobs *et al.* 1999).

7.5 **Benefits of testosterone replacement therapy**

The aim of TRT is to reverse hypogonadal signs and symptoms and enable normal function of androgen-dependent pathways. A subjective response with improved energy, relief of depressive symptoms, regained sexual function, and improved physical and psychological capacity may give the patient a feeling of reclaiming their life. However, more subtle changes perceived by the patient may also be evident and signs of improved glucose metabolism, cardiovascular function, and bone strength may also occur.

Key references

Arver S, *et al.* (1997). Long-term efficacy and safety of a permeation-enhanced testosterone transdermal system in hypogonadal men. *Clin Endocrinol (Oxf)* **47(6)**: 727–37.

Bhasin S, *et al.* (2006). Testosterone therapy in adult men with androgen deficiency syndromes: an endocrine society clinical practice guideline. *J Clin Endocrinol Metab* **91(6)**: 1995–2010.

Dobs AS, et al. (1999). Pharmacokinetics, efficacy, and safety of a permeation-enhanced testosterone transdermal system in comparison with bi-weekly injections of testosterone enanthate for the treatment of hypogonadal men. *J Clin Endocrinol Metab* **84(10)**: 3469–78.

(2001). Men, A.P.o.T.R.i, Report of the National Institute on Aging Advisory Panel on Testosterone Replacement in Men. *J Clin Endocrinol Metab* **86**: 4611–17.

Nieschlag E, et al. (1999). Repeated intramuscular injections of testosterone undecanoate for substitution therapy in hypogonadal men. *Clin Endocrinol (Oxf)* **51(6)**: 757–63.

Nieschlag E, et al. (2004). Testosterone replacement therapy: current trends and future directions. *Hum Reprod Update* **10(5)**: 409–19.

Nieschlag E, et al. (2005). Investigation, treatment and monitoring of late-onset hypogonadism in males. *Aging Male* **8(2)**: 56–8.

Ross RJ, et al. (2004). Pharmacokinetics and tolerability of a bioadhesive buccal testosterone tablet in hypogonadal men. *Eur J Endocrinol* **150**: 57–63.

Sakhri S, Gooren LJ. (2007). Safety aspects of androgen treatment with 5alpha-dihydrotestosterone. *Andrologia* **39(6)**: 216–22.

Wang C, et al. (2004). Long-term testosterone gel (AndroGel) treatment maintains beneficial effects on sexual function and mood, lean and fat mass, and bone mineral density in hypogonadal men. *J Clin Endocrinol Metab* **89(5)**: 2085–98.

Zitzmann M, Nieschlag E. (2007). Androgen receptor gene CAG repeat length and body mass index modulate the safety of long-term intramuscular testosterone undecanoate therapy in hypogonadal men. *J Clin Endocrinol Metab* **92(10)**: 3844–53.

Chapter 8

The prostate and other safety issues

Hermann M. Behre

Key points

- Conditions in which testosterone administration is associated with a high risk of adverse outcome have to be ruled out carefully before initiating therapy.
- Hypogonadal patients on testosterone substitution therapy should be monitored for potential adverse side-effects on a regular basis.
- Testosterone therapy stimulates prostate growth in patients with hypogonadism but only to that comparable with age-matched controls. Patients with lower urinary tract symptoms before as well as during testosterone therapy should obtain a urological evaluation.
- Testosterone therapy is contraindicated in men with prostate carcinoma. However, there is no convincing evidence that testosterone substitution therapy induces prostate carcinoma. Before long-term large prospective studies on the effects of testosterone therapy on prostate function are available, close monitoring of prostate function including digital rectal examination and measurement of prostate-specific antigen is recommended.
- Erythropoiesis is stimulated by testosterone therapy. In patients with haematocrit elevated to the supraphysio-logical range, dose adjustments or cessation of therapy might be indicated.
- In the case of formulation-specific adverse side-effects patients might be switched to another testosterone preparation.

8.1 **Introduction**

The beneficial effects of testosterone therapy in hypogonadal men have to be weighed against potential adverse side-effects. To minimize safety concerns, (1) conditions in which testosterone administration is associated with a high risk of adverse outcome, and (2) contraindications for testosterone administration have to be ruled out carefully before initiating treatment (Tables 8.1 and 8.2). The analysis of randomized controlled trials in men aged ≥45 years who were on testosterone replacement therapy for at least 90 days did not reveal a significant increase in the International Prostate Symptom Score (IPSS) or a higher event rate of urinary retention during treatment.

8.2 **Prostate function**

Androgens are necessary for the development and normal function of the prostate. Major concerns regarding the risks of testosterone therapy have focused primarily on the hyperstimulation of prostate growth and the induction of prostate carcinoma.

8.2.1 **Prostate volume**

As demonstrated in a cross-sectional study, prostate size is significantly smaller in untreated hypogonadal men compared with age-matched control men with normal testosterone levels. Hypogonadal men who have undergone at least 6 months of testosterone replacement therapy have a prostate size comparable with age-matched control men. Similarly, serum levels of prostate-specific antigen (PSA) are not different between age-matched control men and hypogonadal patients on long-term testosterone therapy, and no difference in uroflow parameters can be detected (see Figures 8.1 and 8.2). These data demonstrate that testosterone therapy of hypogonadal men stimulates prostate growth, but only to levels that are seen in age-matched controls. In addition, it has been shown in a longitudinal study that prostate growth per year and final prostate size during long-term testosterone therapy are significantly influenced by androgen receptor gene polymorphism.

The physiological stimulation of prostate growth induced by testosterone therapy might lead to adverse prostate problems in certain circumstances. This could arise in previously untreated patients with hypogonadism who have pre-existing severe symptoms of lower urinary tract obstruction, shown by high IPSS scores or respective

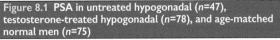

Figure 8.1 PSA in untreated hypogonadal (*n*=47), testosterone-treated hypogonadal (*n*=78), and age-matched normal men (*n*=75)

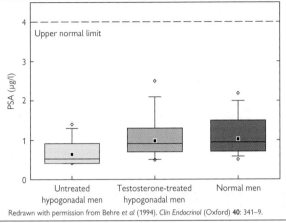

Redrawn with permission from Behre *et al* (1994). *Clin Endocrinol* (Oxford) **40**: 341–9.

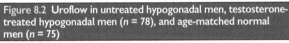

Figure 8.2 Uroflow in untreated hypogonadal men, testosterone-treated hypogonadal men (*n* = 78), and age-matched normal men (*n* = 75)

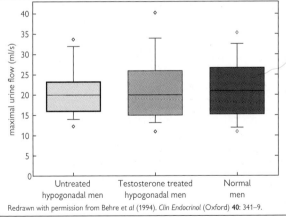

Redrawn with permission from Behre *et al* (1994). *Clin Endocrinol* (Oxford) **40**: 341–9.

clinical findings. These patients should be treated accordingly before testosterone administration (Table 8.2). If patients develop lower urinary tract symptoms, including symptoms of urinary obstruction, during ongoing testosterone therapy this should be an indication for urological evaluation (Table 8.3). The analysis of randomized controlled trials in men aged ≥45 years who were on testosterone replacement therapy for at least 90 days did not reveal a significant increase in the IPSS or a higher event rate of urinary retention during treatment.

8.2.2 Prostate cancer

The regression of prostate cancer after androgen deprivation is well recognized and indicates that many prostate cancer cells, at least initially, are androgen-dependent. Therefore, an existing prostate carcinoma is regarded as an absolute contraindication for testosterone replacement therapy (Tables 8.1 and 8.2).

Table 8.1 Conditions in which testosterone administration is associated with a high risk of adverse outcome and in which testosterone should not be administered: Endocrine Society Clinical Practice Guidelines

Very high risk of serious adverse outcomes
- Metastatic prostate cancer
- Breast cancer

Moderate to high risk of adverse outcomes
- Undiagnosed prostate nodule or induration
- Unexplained PSA elevation
- Erythrocytosis (haematocrit >50%)
- Severe lower urinary tract symptoms associated with benign prostatic hypertrophy as indicated by an American Urological Association prostate symptom score or IPSS >19
- Unstable severe congestive heart failure (class III or IV)

Table 8.2 Contraindications of testosterone therapy in patients with late-onset hypogonadism: current ISA, ISSAM, and EAU recommendations

- Testosterone administration is absolutely contraindicated in men suspected of or having carcinoma of the prostate or breast.
- Men with significant polycythaemia, untreated sleep apnoea, severe heart failure, severe symptoms of lower urinary tract obstruction evident by high scores in the IPSS or clinical findings of bladder outflow obstruction (increased post-micturition residual volume, decreased peak urinary flow, pathological pressure flow-studies) due to an enlarged, clinically benign prostate should not be treated with testosterone. Moderate obstruction represents a partial contraindication. After successful treatment of the obstruction, the contraindication is lifted.
- In the absence of definite contraindications, age as such is not a contraindication to initiate testosterone substitution.

Despite their involvement in prostate growth, the role of androgens in the initiation of prostate cancer is not fully understood. A series of genetic and phenotypic alterations are involved in the multistep nature of prostate carcinogenesis. There are numerous inconsistent reports from the literature indicating that testosterone levels in patients with prostate cancer can be elevated, unchanged, or reduced. Epidemiological investigations have failed to demonstrate consistently that circulating levels of sex hormones are implicated in the aetiology of prostate cancer. However, it should be noted that the negative results of some epidemiological studies could be due to their relatively small size or lack of adjustment for confounding factors.

Recently, a collaborative analysis of the existing worldwide epidemiological data on the associations between endogenous sex hormones and prostate cancer has been performed. Data on serum concentrations of sex hormones from 3886 men with prostate cancer and 6438 control subjects from 18 prospective studies were pooled and the relative risks calculated. No association was found between the risk of prostate cancer and serum concentrations of testosterone, calculated free testosterone, dihydrotestosterone, dehydroepiandrosterone sulphate, androstenedione, androstanediol glucuronide, oestradiol, or calculated free oestradiol. Only the serum concentration of sex hormone binding globulin was modestly inversely associated with prostate cancer risk.

The recent meta-analysis of randomized controlled trials on testosterone therapy in men aged ≥45 years involving 651 men treated with testosterone and 433 with placebo did not reveal an increased incidence of significant PSA elevations or prostate cancers; although prostate biopsies have been performed more often in the testosterone-treated men.

These studies do not provide evidence that testosterone administration to hypogonadal men will induce prostate carcinoma. However, the Institute of Medicine Report on Testosterone and Ageing calculated that a randomized trial with 90% power to detect a 50% increase in the incidence rate of prostate cancer would require 10,000 subjects and take 12.9 years to complete. A comparable study has not been undertaken up to now and, therefore, until final evidence becomes available men treated with testosterone should be monitored carefully by trained physicians for side-effects on the prostate.

A significant number of older men with low testosterone levels have foci of prostate carcinoma, despite normal PSA levels and normal digital rectal examination. It has been suggested that patients with histological prostate cancer and initial normal PSA levels will respond to testosterone therapy with a significantly higher increase of PSA than healthy men. For this reason, close monitoring of PSA levels at the start of treatment is recommended, followed by regular controls, including rectal palpation and PSA measurements during long-term testosterone therapy.

The current Endocrine Society Clinical Practice Guidelines on testosterone therapy of hypogonadal men recommend performing digital rectal examination and checking PSA level before initiating testosterone treatment, at 3 months, and then in accordance with guidelines for prostate cancer screening depending on the age and race of the patient. The indications for obtaining a urological consultation during testosterone therapy are listed in Table 8.3.

Current recommendations of the International Society of Andrology (ISA), the International Society for the Study of the Aging Male (ISSAM), and the European Association of Urology (EAU) on the treatment and monitoring of late-onset hypogonadism regard digital rectal examination and determination of serum PSA in men over the age of 45 years as mandatory at baseline prior to therapy with testosterone, at quarterly intervals for the first 12 months and yearly thereafter. Transrectal ultrasound-guided biopsies of the prostate are considered to be indicated only if the digital rectal examination or serum PSA levels are abnormal.

There is an ongoing discussion about testosterone therapy in men who have been successfully treated for prostate cancer and suffering from confirmed symptomatic hypogonadism. Today, no reliable evidence exists in favour of or against testosterone therapy in these men. According to the current ISA, ISSAM, and EAU recommendations, testosterone therapy might be considered after a prudent interval following successful prostate cancer treatment and if there is no evidence of residual prostate cancer. Therapy should only be initiated if the risks and benefits are clearly understood by the patient. Follow-up has to be particularly careful, and the responsible physician must exercise good clinical judgement together with adequate knowledge of the advantages and disadvantages of testosterone therapy in this situation.

Table 8.3 Indications for obtaining a urological consultation during testosterone therapy: Endocrine Society Clinical Practice Guidelines

- Verified serum PSA concentration >4.0 ng/ml
- Increase in serum PSA concentration >1.4 ng/ml within any 12-month period of testosterone treatment
- PSA velocity of >0.4 ng/ml × year using the PSA level after 6 months of testosterone administration as the reference (only applicable if PSA data are available for a period exceeding 2 years)
- Detection of a prostatic abnormality on digital rectal examination
- American Urological Association prostate symptom score or IPSS >19

8.3 **Erythropoiesis**

Testosterone stimulates erythropoiesis via several mechanisms involving increased erythropoietin secretion and promoting differentiation of erythroid progenitor cells of the bone marrow. While this stimulation is beneficial in many patients with hypogonadism presenting with anaemia before the start of testosterone therapy, an increase of the haematocrit to the supraphysiological range might lead to increased blood viscosity and could be a risk factor for cerebral ischaemia.

Comparative studies have shown that an increased haematocrit is more probable in hypogonadal patients treated with testosterone preparations leading to supraphysiological serum levels of testosterone. The recent meta-analysis of randomized placebo-controlled trials on testosterone therapy in men aged ≥45 years revealed that testosterone-treated men were 3.7 times more likely than placebo-treated men to experience haematocrit greater than 50%. Recently, it has been demonstrated that during long-term treatment with intramuscular testosterone undecanoate a significantly increased haematocrit can be predicted by higher serum levels of testosterone as well as a higher sensitivity of the androgen receptor due to a lower number of CAG repeats of the androgen receptor gene.

The Endocrine Society Clinical Practice Guidelines on testosterone therapy of hypogonadal men recommend against starting testosterone therapy in patients with a haematocrit >50%. During testosterone therapy haematocrit should be determined at baseline, at 3 months, and then annually. If haematocrit is >54%, therapy should be stopped until haematocrit decreases to a safe level. The patient should be evaluated for hypoxia and sleep apnoea, and testosterone therapy reintroduced at a reduced dose.

The current ISA, ISSAM, and EAU recommendations propose periodic haematological assessment before initiation of testosterone treatment, 3-monthly for 1 year, and then annually. In case of elevated haematocrit, appropriate dose adjustments are recommended.

8.4 **Other safety issues**

Testosterone administration might be associated with various other safety issues. The prescribing information and the summary of product characteristics of the respective testosterone formulation used should be consulted for rare potential adverse side-effects not mentioned here.

8.4.1 **Skin and hair**

Testosterone substitution therapy of hypogonadal men can cause significantly increased sebum production, oiliness of skin and, in predisposed men, acne. Adverse effects are seen more often in men treated with preparations leading to supraphysiological serum levels of testosterone. In predisposed hypogonadal men testosterone substitution can lead to male pattern balding. Patients should be informed about these potential side-effects before initiating testosterone therapy.

8.4.2 **Gynaecomastia**

Gynaecomastia can be a sign of hypogonadism and is often seen in untreated patients with Klinefelter's Syndrome. On the other hand breast tenderness and gynaecomastia are potential side-effects of testosterone therapy. However, with modern preparations leading to physiological serum levels of testosterone, gynaecomastia induced by substitution therapy can be considered as an uncommon adverse side-effect.

8.4.3 **Cardiovascular system**

The effects of testosterone therapy on the cardiovascular system as well as on the risk factors for cardiovascular disease are described in detail in Chapter 12. The most comprehensive meta-analysis of randomized placebo-controlled trials on testosterone therapy in men aged ≥45 years did not reveal an increased cardiovascular risk in men treated with testosterone compared with placebo.

8.4.4 **Sleep apnoea**

Early reports suggest that sleep apnoea is a potential adverse side-effect of testosterone therapy. The Endocrine Society Clinical Practice Guidelines recommend against starting testosterone treatment in men with untreated sleep apnoea. The recent meta-analysis of randomized placebo-controlled trials on testosterone therapy in men aged ≥45 years did not reveal an increased frequency of men with a new diagnosis of sleep apnoea during testosterone treatment.

8.4.5 **Suppression of spermatogenesis**

In hypogonadal patients with adequate spermatogenesis, testosterone therapy can suppress sperm production via suppression of gonadotrophins and lead to infertility. Decreased sperm production can be associated with a decrease of testicular volume. Various studies have shown that this effect of testosterone administration on gonadotrophin secretion, spermatogenesis, and testicular volume is reversible upon cessation of therapy.

8.4.6 **Formulation-specific safety issues**

In addition to the above-mentioned safety issues, the various testosterone preparations currently available for substitution therapy might have formulation-specific adverse side-effects and safety concerns. Testosterone pellet implants can lead to infections, bruising, and extrusion at the implantation site. Intramuscular testosterone esters might cause pain, subcutaneous haematoma, and, rarely, infections at the injection site. Oral testosterone preparations can lead to a decrease in cholesterol serum levels and – in the case of administration of the obsolete methyl-testosterone – to impaired liver function and hepato-toxicity.

Skin reactions such as redness and itching are observed after administration of certain testosterone patches available for transder-mal therapy. Patients treated with transdermal testosterone gel have to be informed about the potential risk of testosterone transfer to the partner or children upon close contact. These patients need to be reminded to cover application sites with clothing and to wash skin at the application site and hands with soap before having skin-to-skin contact with another person. Buccal testosterone tablets might cause alterations in taste or gum irritation.

The treating physicians as well as the patients are advised to consult the prescribing information and summary of product characteristics of the respective testosterone preparation for formulation-specific incidence and severity of adverse side-effects. In case of formulation-specific adverse side-effects patients might be switched to another testosterone preparation.

8.5 Conclusions

Several decades of testosterone substitution treatment of hypogo-nadal men have shown that this therapy can be considered as com-parably safe. This only holds true if contraindications for testosterone therapy, such as existing prostate or breast cancer, are ruled out and patients with increased risk for adverse side-effects are carefully evaluated and treated appropriately before starting testosterone therapy. Long-term monitoring of testosterone therapy on a regular basis according to the most recent national and/or international treatment recommendations is mandatory.

Key references

Behre HM, Bohmeyer J, Nieschlag E. (1994). Prostate volume in testos-terone-treated and untreated hypogonadal men in comparison to age-matched normal controls. *Clin Endocrinol (Oxf)* **40**: 341–9.

Bhasin S, Cunningham GR, Hayes FJ, Matsumoto AM, Snyder PJ, Swerdloff RS, Montori VM. (2006). Testosterone therapy in adult men with androgen deficiency syndromes: an Endocrine Society Clinical Practice Guideline. *J Clin Endocrinol Metab* **91**: 1995–2010.

Calof OM, Singh AB, Lee ML, Kenny AM, Urban RJ, Tenover JL, Bhasin S. (2005). Adverse events associated with testosterone replacement in middle-aged and older men: a meta-analysis of randomized, placebo-controlled trials. *J Gerontol A Biol Sci Med Sci* **60**: 1451–7.

Endogenous Hormones, Prostate Cancer Collaborative Group, Roddam AW, Allen NE, Appleby P, Key TJ. (2008). Endogenous sex hormones and prostate cancer: a collaborative analysis of 18 prospective studies. *J Natl Cancer Inst* **100**: 170–83.

Liverman CT, Blazer DG (eds). (2004). *Testosterone and aging: clinical research directions*. Institute of Medicine of the National Academies. The National Academies Press, Washington.

Nieschlag E, Behre HM (eds). (2000). *Andrology – male reproductive health and dysfunction*, 2nd edn. Springer-Verlag, Berlin.

Nieschlag E, Behre HM (eds). (2004). *Testosterone – action, deficiency, substitution*, 3rd edn. Cambridge University Press, Cambridge.

Nieschlag E, Swerdloff R, Behre HM, Gooren LJ, Kaufman JM, Legros JJ, Lunenfeld B, Morley JE, Schulman C, Wang C, Weidner W, Wu FC. (2005). Investigation, treatment and monitoring of late-onset hypogonadism in males: ISA, ISSAM, and EAU recommendations. *Eur Urol* **48**: 1–4.

Zitzmann M, Nieschlag E. (2007). Androgen receptor gene CAG repeat length and body mass index modulate the safety of long-term intramuscular testosterone undecanoate therapy in hypogonadal men. *J Clin Endocrinol Metab* **92**: 3844–53.

Zitzmann M, Depenbusch M, Gromoll J, Nieschlag E. (2003). Prostate volume and growth in testosterone-substituted hypogonadal men are dependent on the CAG repeat polymorphism of the androgen receptor gene: a longitudinal pharmacogenetic study. *J Clin Endocrinol Metab* **88**: 2049–54.

Chapter 9

Puberty and fertility

T. Hugh Jones and Richard Quinton

> **Key points**
> - Testosterone therapy improves psychosocial well-being and peak bone mass in constitutional delayed puberty.
> - Testosterone therapy for failure of puberty due to permanent hypogonadism is essential for timely pubertal development to reduce the risk of psychosocial and psychosexual stresses.
> - Spermatogenesis can be induced or enhanced in a high proportion of men with secondary hypogonadism with gonadotrophin therapy.
> - The management of delayed or failed puberty and fertility is complex and should only be dealt with by experienced specialist clinicians.

9.1 Causes of delayed puberty

9.1.1 Constitutional delayed puberty

This is defined as a delay in onset of pubertal development significantly beyond that of the peer group. It is associated with a retardation of the rate of linear growth as well as the timing of progression to develop secondary sexual characteristics. There may be a family history of the father, mother, brother, or sister also being a late developer. The condition can lead to psychological pressures from the peer group leading to social stresses and family concern. Chronological bone age can be assessed by hand X-rays using appropriate charts. A significantly younger chronological than actual age, supports the diagnosis of delayed puberty in the absence of other conditions that would cause disparity. Constitutional delayed puberty is a transient state of hypogonadotrophic hypogonadism with low levels of gonadotrophins and testosterone. If left untreated all will eventually pass through puberty. In the past, treatment has been indicated if there is a state of psychological stress. Evidence, however, has shown that there is also a benefit of treatment on bone mineral density and on body composition.

9.1.2 **Permanent hypogonadism**

Permanent hypogonadism is failure of puberty caused by a genetic or acquired form of either primary or secondary hypogonadism. These conditions such as Klinefelter's Syndrome and Kallmann's Syndrome are discussed in Chapters 4 and 5. A genetic or acquired form of secondary hypogonadism before the age of 11 years is usually associated with a testicular size of <4 ml. Some causes of primary hypogonadism, such as Klinefelter's Syndrome can stimulate tallness due to failure of the epiphyses to close.

If individuals present with failed puberty after the age of 18 years it is almost certain that they have permanent hypogonadism. Many may not present until their early twenties or even until their sixties.

9.2 **Management of delayed puberty**

In the absence of a diagnosis of a cause of permanent hypogonadism, individuals are treated as constitutional delayed puberty. There should, however, be continuous clinical surveillance so that the cause of permanent hypogonadism may eventually become apparent.

The treatment of choice over recent years has been the use of the injectable forms of testosterone esters. In the UK mixed esters (i.e. Sustanon®100 containing testosterone propionate 20 mg, phenylpropionate 40 mg and isocaproate 40 mg or Sustanon®250 with testosterone propionate 30 mg, phenylpropionate 60 mg, isocaproate 60 mg, and decanoate 100 mg) are used and in other countries testosterone enanthate or cypionate are used. Oral therapy may also be used but as described in Chapter 7 it has low bioavailability. The newer formulations of testosterone gels may be suitable for subjects with needle phobias; however, there have been no publications reporting their use in the management of delayed puberty.

It is standard practice that the testosterone is initiated at low doses, gradually increasing over a period of time to full adult doses especially in cases of permanent hypogonadism. Suggested regimens are as follows.

9.2.1 **Constitutional delayed puberty**

Treatment is usually initiated with a testosterone ester dose of 50–100 mg monthly for the first 3 months depending on the age and height at presentation (use lower doses in younger boys and in older boys with short stature to avoid early closure of the epiphyses). After 3 months the patient is reviewed for physiological changes such as increases in testicular size and endogenous testosterone production (assessed by a testosterone level before the third injection). If there is benefit then the same dose is continued, if not then the dose is increased by 25–50 mg for a further 3 months before being re-evaluated.

An increase in testicular size is the key factor that will determine whether the individual has constitutional delayed puberty and not a permanent form of hypogonadism. If there is testicular enlargement and once the individual has caught up with his peers in the development of secondary sexual characteristics then treatment can be stopped. It is prudent to re-check luteinizing hormone (LH), follicle-stimulating hormone (FSH), and testosterone levels 6 months later to be sure that he has attained normal post-pubertal production levels.

9.2.2 **Permanent hypogonadism**

This group comprises two types of presentation: those diagnosed with a permanent cause of hypogonadism and those initially treated as constitutional delayed puberty, in whom it becomes clearer at a later date that they have a permanent hypogonadism. Initially, in boys under the age of 16 years (at the discretion of the clinician) the treatment is the same as that of constitutional delayed puberty. After 16 years the dose is gradually increased to that of the adult replacement level of testosterone esters 200 mg twice monthly. At that stage the individual's treatment can be converted to a testosterone replacement therapy mode of his choice. Most will chose the 3-monthly depot injection of testosterone undecanoate. This is better for convenience and compliance.

In conditions such as Klinefelter's, testosterone deficiency is associated with gaining excessive height. A more rapid and earlier increase in testosterone dose may be required to retard linear growth by inducing earlier closure of the epiphyses.

9.2.3 **Gonadotrophin therapy**

In permanent forms of secondary hypogonadism either gonadotrophin-releasing hormone (GnRH) pulsatile therapy or human chorionic gonadotrophin (hCG) therapy alone or in combination with FSH can be used to induce puberty. Pulsatile GnRH therapy is expensive and not usually practical in the management of puberty. hCG is not produced by men but when given pharmacologically it has an LH-like action on the testis. The dose of hCG can be introduced at 500 units twice weekly, gradually increasing to attain adult levels as described below.

A small testicular size can have major effects on psychosexual confidence leading to anxiety and stress. Failure of testicular development is usually associated with secondary hypogonadism with pre-pubertal onset. The failure of testicular growth is particularly pronounced (<4 ml) in congenital forms of hypogonadotrophic hypogonadism, which includes Kallmann's Syndrome and idiopathic hypogonadotrophic hypogonadism. FSH has the main trophic effect on the testes with LH having a much smaller action.

Combined hCG and FSH treatment in men with these disorders can significantly increase testicular size to acceptable levels in some men over a period of 6–12 months (Figure 9.1). Testosterone levels should first be normalized by administering hCG, commencing at a dose of 500 units subcutaneously self-administered twice weekly. The dose is then increased after 2 months to 1000 units twice weekly then by 1000 units twice weekly every 2 months until a testosterone level within the normal range is achieved (ideally above 15 nmol/l). hCG can stimulate oestradiol levels which need to be monitored to be sure that the levels do not significantly exceed the male normal range.

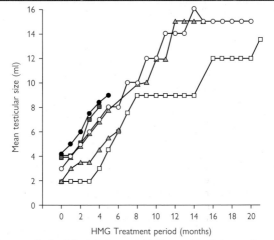

Figure 9.1 Effect of FSH (in form of hMG) on mean testicular size in males with genetic causes of secondary hypogonadism

Young men with either Kallman's Syndrome or isolated hypogonadotrophic hypogonadism were treated with combined hMG (human menopausal gonadotrophin containing FSH and LH) and hCG to stimulate spermatogenesis and increase testicular size. All subjects had a mean testicular size of ≤ 4 ml with complete gonadotrophin deficiency. hCG was given and dose adjusted to give normal testosterone levels prior to commencing hMG. Redrawn with permission from Jones, T. H. *et al* (1993). *Clin Endocrinol* (Oxford), **38**: 203–8.

FSH (available as recombinant or highly purified urinary preparations) is then added at a dose of 150 units administered subcutaneously thrice weekly. Testicular size is monitored and once either a reasonable size, e.g. 10–15 ml is achieved, the growth plateaus, or if after 6 months the testes has not responded, then treatment is stopped. The testis may become softer but a reasonable size is usually maintained. This form of therapy can be expensive.

9.3 **Fertility**

Male hypogonadism is effectively associated with subfertility due to impaired or absent spermatogenesis. Where the sperm count and/or quality is inadequate for 'natural' impregnation, treatment options are typically restricted to ICSI (if sperm can be retrieved from either the ejaculate or testicular aspirate) and donor sperm insemination. Testosterone therapy has no place in the management of these patients and indeed can suppress spermatogenesis.

A notable exception to this is secondary hypogonadism, where azoospermia or oligospermia normally responds well to sustained therapy with either gonadotrophins or pulsatile GnRH. Good prognostic indicators include: the presence of sperm in the ejaculate pre-treatment; onset of secondary hypogonadism in adult life rather than pre-puberty; larger baseline testicular volume and normally descended scrotal testes. Where congenital secondary hypogonadism is associated with a history of bilateral testicular maldescent, corrected after age 8–10, and testes are of abnormally firm consistency with volumes under 4 ml, the pre-treatment probability of successful spermatogenesis induction is exceedingly low.

Normal spermatogenesis requires the simultaneous action of (1) FSH to promote germ cell proliferation and Sertoli cell function, and (2) LH to promote germ cell differentiation and stimulate testosterone synthesis and secretion by Leydig cells. The degree of prior exposure to endogenous or exogenous FSH is also contributory; hence, men with adult-onset secondary hypogonadism respond faster and better to spermatogenesis-induction therapy than those with secondary hypogonadism of prepubertal onset.

The overall hormone replacement therapy of men with a broader hypopituitarism should first be optimized before commencing gonadotrophin therapy for the initiation or enhancement of spermatogenesis. Moreover, as a minimum requirement, details of the age, body mass index, and menstrual history of the female partner should be obtained and, if there is the least doubt, a formal (referral for) assessment should be made of her ovulatory reserve, tubal patency, Rubella serology, etc. Finally, if secondary hypogonadism appears to be genetic in origin, e.g. as part of KS or CPHD the couple need to be made aware that it might be inherited by their offspring.

For adult-onset secondary hypogonadism, androgen replacement is simply discontinued and the patient taught to self-inject hCG instead. The optimal treatment dose is subject to interindividual variation, ranging from 1000 to 15,000 units/week divided into two or three subcutaneous injections; however, a reasonable starting dose would be 2000 units twice weekly. The dose is then titrated at intervals of 2–3 months, guided by serum levels of total testosterone, calculated free testosterone, and oestradiol; dose adjustments are made to maintain all three parameters within their respective reference ranges. This regimen is no more expensive than many forms of direct androgen replacement therapy and tends to better preserve testicular volume (so that some men may choose to continue on it as a long-term treatment option); it may be sufficient by itself to re-awaken or augment spermatogenesis. This, however, generally only occurs in men who developed their hypogonadism after a normal puberty.

If there is insufficient response after 4–6 months, FSH should be added at a standard dose of 150 units three times a week, injected subcutaneously by self-administration. It can take between 2 and 18 months to stimulate spermatogenesis to an appropriate level to be able to achieve conception. If conception does not occur reasonably soon after normal spermatogenesis is established, the couple will need guidance in evaluating the relative financial and/or personal implications of continuing with attempts to conceive 'naturally', versus moving down the 'assisted conception' pathway. With sufficient sperm frozen and stored pending ICSI, the patient can potentially resume his previous testosterone replacement regimen (or remain on hCG alone).

Secondary hypogonadism of prebubertal onset typically takes longer to respond and treatment occasionally needs to be prolonged for over 2 years before sperm first appear in the ejaculate (though 4–9 months would be a more typical period). It may then take another 6–12 months of treatment before peak spermatogenesis is achieved. Men with congenital secondary hypogonadism may have a relatively sluggish spermatogenetic response; this may be because they did not undergo previous gonadotrophin – driven bursts of germ cell proliferation during the neonatal and pubertal periods. Men with combined secondary hypogonadism and growth hormone deficiency who consistently fail to initiate spermatogenesis should be considered for concomitant growth hormone replacement therapy before assuming that treatment has failed. Growth hormone has been shown to play a key role in spermatogenesis.

Restoration of endogenous gonadotrophin secretion with GnRH, using a programmable minipump to deliver pulses 2 h apart via an indwelling subcutaneous cannula; it offers the most elegant and physiological form of treatment, with any hitherto unsuspected defects of testicular function becoming manifest through disproportionate rises in FSH levels. However, as it is no more effective than conventional gonadotrophin therapy, its use in men tends to be restricted to centres with long-standing research interests in the physiology of human gonadotrophin secretion.

For a man with testes volume of <5 ml and no history of cryptorchidism the pre-treatment probability of achieving normal spermatogenesis is about 60%, with an additional 20% chance of achieving a count adequate for ICSI. As with any couple, of course, having a normal sperm count gives no guarantee of successful conception; by contrast there are reliable reports of men with secondary hypogonadism who successfully impregnate their partners with counts <5.0 × 106 motile sperm/ml.

Rather than starting hCG and FSH therapy simultaneously, there are good theoretical reasons for initially just adding FSH 75 units thrice weekly to the patient's existing direct androgen replacement regimen for a period of months; the aim being to promote a phase of pure germ cell proliferation, before the onset of hCG-induced germ cell differentiation.

When testicular volume has normalized, but the ejaculate remains azoospermic, the possibility of obstructive tubulopathy should be actively investigated. A history of sexually transmitted disease or positive Chlamydia serology are both highly suggestive (particularly if serum levels of the Sertoli cell-derived peptides, hormones anti-Mullerian hormone (AMH) or Inhibin B, are normal); however definitive proof resides in testicular aspiration, which may also provide a therapeutic solution in conjunction with sperm storage and ICSI.

Practical problems for the patient and physician include (1) the absence of a specific product licence for male hypogonadotrophic infertility for many gonadotrophin preparations and, frequently, (2) the lack of a defined budget for the supply or reimbursement of gonadotrophin ampoules in this context. Such issues are typically more easily addressed when the endocrinologist or clinical andrologist works closely with his/her local reproductive gynaecology colleague(s). In addition, patients may be concerned at the prospect of injecting products derived from pooled female human urine (menopausal for FSH and pregnant for hCG). Nevertheless, after several decades of use they can be reassured of the complete absence of any evidence for prion disease transmission.

Key references

Büchter D, Behre HM, Kliesch S, Nieschlag E. (1998). Pulsatile GnRH or human chorionic gonadotropin/human menopausal gonadotropin as effective treatment for men with hypogonadotropic hypogonadism: a review of 42 cases. *Eur J Endocrinol* **139**: 298–303.

Jones TH, Darne JF. (1993). Self-administered subcutaneous human menopausal gonadotrophin for the stimulation of testicular growth and the initiation of spermatogenesis in hypogonadotrophic hypogonadism. *Clin Endocrinol* **38**: 203–8.

Jones TH, Darne JF, McGarrigle H. (1994). Diurnal rhythm of testosterone induced by twice weekly HCG therapy in isolated hypogonadotrophic hypogonadism: a comparison between subcutaneous and intramuscular HCG administration. *Eur J Endocrinol* **131**: 173–8.

Nachtigall LB, Boepple PA, Pralong FP, Crowley WF Jr. (1997). Adult-onset idiopathic hypogonadotropic hypogonadism – a treatable form of male infertility. *N Engl J Med* **336**: 410–15.

Richmond EJ, Rogol AD. (2007). Male pubertal development and the role of androgen therapy. *Nat Clin Pract* **3**: 338–434.

Chapter 10

Testosterone and erectile dysfunction

Aksam A. Yassin, Ahmed I. El-Sakka, and Farid Saad

Key points

- Severe hypogonadism in men usually results in loss of libido and potency, which can be restored by androgen administration.
- The original insights into the mechanisms of action of androgens on sexual function indicated that androgens mainly exert effects on libido.
- Testosterone appears to have profound effects on tissues of the penis involved in the mechanism of erection.
- Testosterone deficiency impairs the anatomical and physiological/biochemical substrate of erectile capacity, which is reversible upon androgen treatment.
- Androgen deprivation in humans results in low sexual desire or libido, impaired erectile function and alteration in penile composition and size.
- The administration of phosphodiesterase type 5 inhibitors is not always sufficient to restore erectile potency, and the administration of testosterone improves the therapeutic response of these inhibitors considerably.
- Low levels of testosterone are closely related to manifestations of other aetiological factors in erectile dysfunction, such as atherosclerotic disease and diabetes mellitus.

10.1 Testosterone and erectile function

10.1.1 The role of testosterone in male sexual functioning

This chapter will focus on the role of testosterone in erectile function and dysfunction (ED). Systematic observations on testosterone (pathophysiology) were carried out when testosterone became pharmaceutically available in the middle of the twentieth century. The early investigations pointed to a prominent role of testosterone in sexual interest while the effects of testosterone on erectile function were less appreciated. The view of many practitioners was that treatment of ED with testosterone was not very efficacious. Then, in 1998 a new class of drugs, the phosphodiesterase type 5 (PDE-5) inhibitors, was introduced. These highly efficacious and relatively safe compounds have had a profound impact on the diagnosis and treatment of ED. Once mainly the domain of the urologist attempting to define its precise aetiology, ED is now largely treated by first-line primary care physicians or GPs, usually without an elaborate diagnostic work-up; however, they have had a good degree of success. Despite the simplicity and safety of the present therapy of ED with PDE-5 inhibitors, approximately 50% of patients discontinue treatment.

10.1.2 Recent insights into the significance of testosterone for male health

In recent years there has been renewed interest in the role of testosterone in male (patho)physiology in a broader sense, and more significantly the place of testosterone in ED. Recent studies provide convincing evidence that testosterone has a powerful effect on the anatomy and physiology of penile erection. Furthermore, it has become clear that testosterone is not simply just one of the many factors playing a part in erectile (dys)function. Circulating levels of testosterone are closely related to the manifestations of other aetiological factors in ED, such as atherosclerotic disease and diabetes mellitus (Figure 10.1). The latter are components of the metabolic syndrome, which is correlated with lower-than-normal testosterone levels. Therefore, the role of testosterone in erectile (dys)function is increasingly recognized. In patients with ED a decline in testosterone levels was found over a 4-year follow-up period. The proportion of men with ED and low testosterone levels varies between studies, but is about 20%. In a large population-based cohort of older men, an association between total testosterone, bioavailable testosterone, free testosterone, sexual hormone-binding globulin, and ED could be established. Testosterone levels were associated with a decrease in risk of ED only in men with increased luteinizing hormone levels. These findings have potential implications for the diagnosis of hypogonadism if testosterone levels are borderline, and may possibly lead to individualization of androgen therapies in men. This was confirmed in a clinical study where men responded favourably to testosterone treatment when their testosterone levels were low but still in the normal range.

10.1.3 Erectile dysfunction as a symptom of ill health

Rather than a disease in itself, ED is (particularly in elderly men who have enjoyed normal sexual functions earlier in life) a manifestation of pathologies of the biological systems involved in erectile function

(Figure 10.1). The successful treatment of erectile difficulties, with drugs such as the PDE-5 inhibitors, has led to a concept of erectile failure as an entity in itself rather than an expression of underlying pathology or its constituents.

10.2 Redefining the role of testosterone in erectile function

10.2.1 Effects on sexual motivation

When testosterone became pharmaceutically available, systematic studies were undertaken to define more precisely the role of testosterone in a man's sexual functioning. Most of the information that has been collected is from androgen withdrawal/replacement studies of hypogonadal men. Surprisingly, the findings strongly suggested that it was mainly sexual interest that was androgen dependent. Further, the studies provided evidence that various types of erections showed a different relationship with circulating testosterone. In the first studies spontaneous erections, particularly those that occur during sleep, and probably fantasy-induced erections were thought to be exclusively androgen dependent, whereas erections in response to erotic (e.g. visual or tactile) stimuli were less so. Sexual complaints of patients relate to the latter type of erections, erections in the context of anticipated sexual activity. The original studies, however, monitored only penile circumference but not stiffness; later observations showed that androgens do affect penile responses to erotic stimuli with regard to the duration of response, and maximal degree of rigidity, which are all significant aspects of androgen effects on sexual functioning. Nevertheless, these observations led to the belief that androgens had effects primarily on sexual interest or motivation. The influence

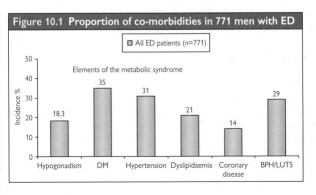

Figure 10.1 Proportion of co-morbidities in 771 men with ED

on the penile erection was thought to be indirect, via the effects on libido, rather than direct on penile tissues. Consequently, it was assumed that androgens were therapeutically not very useful when men complained of erectile difficulties while their sexual desire was not impaired, which was often the reason men seek medical consultation.

10.2.2 Critical levels of testosterone for sexual function

Another reason why testosterone was not regarded as a therapeutic option in men with ED was the finding that the blood level of testosterone critical for restoring sexual interest (though varying between individuals) appeared to be 60–70% of the reference values for eugonadal men. It is of note that these observations were done in men with a wide range of ages and not specifically addressing the issue in older men. Consequently, it was assumed that in men with ED and low-normal or slightly lower than normal androgen levels (common in an elderly population) treatment with testosterone was likely to be of no help. This corresponded with the clinical experience of many practitioners. When the PDE-5 inhibitors were introduced in 1998, patients who had earlier failed treatment with androgens or other types of therapy, could now be successfully treated. The threshold for the biological actions of testosterone might be higher in elderly men compared with young men.

10.3 Testosterone and erectile tissue

Over the last 15 years the age-related decline of circulating testosterone in men has received increasing attention, not only in relation to sexual functioning but also in the wider context of male health. A recent study demonstrated a steady decline in testosterone level throughout a 4-year follow-up period in patients with ED. Moreover, new research has presented convincing evidence, so far mainly in laboratory animals, that (1) testosterone has profound effects on tissues of the penis involved in the mechanism of erection, and (2) testosterone deficiency impairs the anatomical and physiological substrate of erectile capacity. Recent findings demonstrated that restoring normal plasma levels of testosterone is beneficial in the treatment of ED. It has been shown that the full therapeutic potential of PDE-5 inhibitors will only become manifest in a eugonadal state (Figure 10.2). These results changed the earlier concept that the effects of testosterone are primarily and predominantly involved with libidinous aspects of the male, and not directly on the penis as well.

Animal experiments and limited human observations suggest that androgens are necessary to maintain the integrity of the anatomical structures of the penile erectile tissue and, further, that androgens

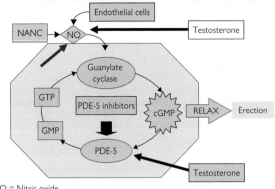

Figure 10.2 PDE-5 inhibitors are less effective in ED patients with testosterone deficiency

NO = Nitric oxide
NANC = Non-adrenergic-noncholinergic neurons
PDE-5 = Phosphodiesterase type 5

Androgens regulate endothelial nitric oxide synthase (eNOS) expression and neural nitric oxide synthase (nNOS) expression activity as well as PDE-5 expression and activity.

are essential to the biochemical mechanisms involved in penile erection. Testosterone deficiency has an adverse effect on cavernosal nerve fibres in the rat model, which improve after testosterone replacement. Also, the effects of castration on peripheral (cavernous nerve) and central (medial preoptic area) stimulation of penile erection have been demonstrated.

10.3.1 Androgen effects on the structural, ultrastructural, and molecular composition of cavernosal tissue

Animal studies have demonstrated that androgen deprivation produces changes in the histological properties of penile structures. In a rat model it could be demonstrated that androgen deprivation leads to loss of elastic fibres in the tunica albuginea and of smooth muscle fibres in the corpus cavernosum, which were replaced by collagenous fibres in both structures; this could lead to impaired erection due to venous reflux (Figure 10.3). Mesenchymal pluripotent cells follow a myogenic lineage or adipogenic lineage depending on circulating levels of testosterone. Even a 50% reduction in circulating testosterone reduced intracavernosal blood pressure, which was not enhanced by administration of the PDE-5 inhibitor vardenafil. Adequate testosterone treatment can restore venous leakage in the corpus cavernosum, which is a frequent aetiological factor in ED in elderly men (Figure 10.4).

Figure 10.3 Veno-occlusive mechanism in penile erection

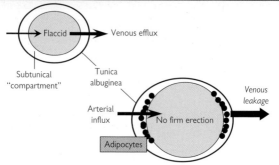

In the flaccid penis, a balance exists between arterial influx and venous efflux. Androgens regulate differentiation of progenitor vascular-stroma cells into myogenic and adipogenic lineages. Testosterone deficiency leads to fat cells accumulation in the subtunical region, resulting in veno-occlusive dysfunction or venous leakage causing reduced strength or failure of the erection.

Figure 10.4 Venous leakage caused by testosterone deficiency

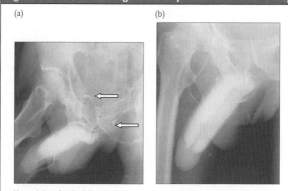

Venous leakage (baseline left) evidenced by cavernosography in a hypogonadal man with erectile dysfunction, and after 4.5 months administration of testosterone undecanoate (right) no venous leak with better penile composition and opacification. Testosterone replacement has restored the veno-occlusive mechanism. Reproduced with permission from Traish AM, Guay AT (2006). *Journal of Sexual Medicine.*

10.4 Testosterone treatment of sexual dysfunction

10.4.1 Effects of testosterone therapy to elderly men with erectile dysfunction

While the effects of testosterone treatment on the parameters of sexual functioning in younger and middle-aged men have been convincing, the effects in elderly men are not easy to demonstrate. As many as 50% of men in an ageing population may benefit from normalization of testosterone levels. The effects may not become apparent before 3 or more months after starting treatment; therefore, it is important not to make judgements too quickly with regard to the efficacy of testosterone treatment. With regard to safety it has been found that neither prostate volume, nor the level of prostate-specific antigen was significantly changed after 1 year of testosterone replacement therapy in patients with hypogonadism associated with ED.

10.4.2 Effects of testosterone treatment in men who would not benefit from treatment with PDE-5 inhibitors

The success rate of treatment with sildenafil in a cohort of 162 men >60 years was only 47%. It could further be established that among the risk factors predicting a poor response to sildenafil were smoking and hypogonadism (plasma testosterone <3 ng/ml; <10.4 nmol/l). In line with this a number of factors (e.g. the circulating levels of free testosterone, independent of age, positively correlated with the degree of relaxation of the corporal smooth muscle cells and the cavernous endothelial cells) support the role of androgens in potentially regulating smooth muscle function and ultimately the enhancement of erection.

There is support for this mechanism of action of testosterone on the erectile tissues of the penis. The effects of androgen administration in 20 patients with arteriogenic ED not responding to treatment with sildenafil 100 mg alone, had been confirmed using dynamic colour duplex ultrasound. The patients' testosterone levels were in the lower quartile of the normal range. In this placebo-controlled study, treatment with transdermal testosterone raised plasma testosterone levels; this led to an increase of arterial inflow into the cavernous tissue and to an improvement of ED thus enhancing the response to treatment with PDE-5 inhibitors. In line with the above it has been documented that normal plasma testosterone is required for erectile function. In severely hypogonadal men (plasma testosterone <2.0 ng/ml; <7 nmol/l) the nocturnal penile tumescence, ultrasound measurement of arterial carvernous inflow, and visually stimulated erection in response to sildenafil 50 mg or apomorphine 3 mg were minimal. The responses to these pharmacological stimuli normalized after 6 months of treatment, with testosterone patches. This provided further evidence for the significant role of normal testosterone levels for the process of erection. Several clinical studies have reported the beneficial effects of the combination of PDE-5 inhibitors with testosterone (Figure 10.5). The notion that testosterone and PDE-5 inhibitors have synergistic effects on nocturnal erections was also confirmed in men in a laboratory setting.

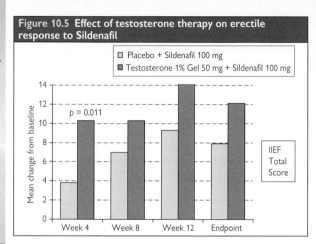

Figure 10.5 Effect of testosterone therapy on erectile response to Sildenafil

☐ Placebo + Sildenafil 100 mg
☐ Testosterone 1% Gel 50 mg + Sildenafil 100 mg

p = 0.011

IIEF Total Score

10.5 New insights into testosterone and erectile dysfunction

The erectile response in animals is centrally and peripherally regulated by androgens. Severe hypogonadism in men usually results in loss of libido and potency, which can be restored by androgen administration.

The original insights into the mechanisms of action of androgens on sexual function indicated that androgens particularly exert effects on libido and that sleep-related erections were androgen sensitive; however, erections in response to erotic stimuli were relatively androgen-independent.

There are a number of recent developments that shed new light on the testosterone treatment of ED in ageing men. There is growing insight that testosterone has profound effects on tissues of the penis involved in the mechanism of erection and that testosterone deficiency impairs the anatomical and physiological/biochemical substrate of erectile capacity, which is reversible after androgen treatment. Several studies have indicated that PDE-5 inhibitors are not always sufficient to restore erectile potency in men, and that testosterone treatment improves the therapeutic response of PDE-5 inhibitors considerably. Therefore, assessment of hormonal profiles, particularly testosterone in all patients with ED could help define the aetiology, and would certainly benefit the treatment of patients with ED and its associated hypogonadism. Incorporation of testosterone in the armamentarium of the diagnosis of ED is presently mandatory. Bioavailable testosterone is a more sensitive test than total testosterone in men with diabetes mellitus. Normalization of testosterone may also have a beneficial effect on the metabolic syndrome. It has been found that the severity of ED correlated inversely with visceral adiposity.

Key references

El-Sakka AI, Hassoba HM. (2006). Patients with erectile. age-related testosterone depletion in dysfunction. *J Urol* **176**: 2589–93.

Gooren LJ, Saad F. (2006). Recent insights into androgen action on the anatomical and physiological substrate of penile erection. *Asian J Androl* **8**: 3–9.

Kapoor D, Clarke SKS, Channer KS, Jones TH. (2007). Erectile dysfunction is associated with low bioactive testosterone levels and visceral adiposity in men with type 2 diabetes. *Int J Androl* **30**: 500–507.

Rochira V, Balestrieri A, et al. (2006). Sildenafil improves sleep-related erections in hypogonadal men: evidence from a randomized, placebo-controlled, crossover study of a synergic role for both testosterone and sildenafil on penile erections. *J Androl* **27**: 165–75.

Shabsigh R, Rajfer J, Aversa A, Traish AM, Yassin A, Kalinchenko SY, Buvat J. (2006). The evolving role of testosterone in the treatment of erectile dysfunction. *Int. J Clin Pract* **60**: 1087–92.

Suzuki N, Sato Y, et al. (2007). Effect of testosterone on intracavernous pressure elicited with electrical stimulation of the medial preoptic area and cavernous nerve in male rats. *J Androl* **28**: 218–22.

Traish AM, Goldstein I, et al. (2007). Testosterone and erectile function: from basic research to a new clinical paradigm for managing men with androgen insufficiency and erectile dysfunction. *Eur Urol* **52**: 54–70.

Traish AM, Guay AT. (2006). Are androgens critical for penile erections in humans? Examining the clinical and preclinical evidence. *J Sex Med* **3**: 382–407.

Yassin A, Saad F. (2006a). Treatment of sexual dysfunction of hypogonadal patients with long-acting testosterone undecanoate (Nebido). *World J Urol* **24**: 639–44.

Yassin AA, Saad F. (2006b). Dramatic improvement of penile venous leakage upon testosterone administration. A case report and review of literature. *Andrologia* **38**: 34–7.

Chapter 11

Obesity, metabolic syndrome, and diabetes

T. Hugh Jones

Key points

- Low testosterone and sex hormone-binding globulin levels in healthy men are independent risk factors for the subsequent development of the metabolic syndrome and type 2 diabetes.
- There is a high prevalence of hypogonadism in men with the metabolic syndrome and type 2 diabetes.
- Low testosterone levels are associated with insulin resistance.
- The Hypogonadal–Obesity–Adipocytokine Cycle Hypothesis defines the stimulatory effect of obesity on testosterone metabolism and the impaired ability of the hypothalamic–pituitary–testicular axis to respond.
- The diagnosis of hypogonadism in men with the metabolic syndrome and diabetes requires rigorous assessment and the decision to treat should be made by an experienced clinician.
- Short-term studies have demonstrated that testosterone replacement improves insulin resistance, glycaemic control, and visceral adiposity.

11.1 Introduction

There is a high prevalence of low testosterone levels in men with: (1) obesity; (2) the metabolic syndrome; and (3) type 2 diabetes. The prevalence of obesity is increasing at dramatic rates throughout the Western World. Visceral obesity is an essential component of the metabolic syndrome, which is a pre-diabetic phase. Visceral adipose tissue is highly metabolically active. The volume of visceral fat is directly proportional to the degree of insulin resistance. Insulin resistance is central to the development of hyperglycaemia, dyslipidaemia, hypertension, endothelial dysfunction, and a pro-thrombotic and pro-inflammatory milieu. Each of these factors independently promotes atherogenesis. It is well known that the metabolic syndrome and type 2 diabetes are associated with a high prevalence of cardiovascular disease. Indeed, 75% of men with type 2 diabetes die from cardiovascular disease.

There is now convincing evidence that there is a higher prevalence of testosterone deficiency in men with the metabolic syndrome and type 2 diabetes. There is also good evidence that men with low testosterone levels, which include non-obese subjects, are at higher risk of developing these conditions. Visceral obesity is an essential component of the metabolic syndrome and an independent risk factor for cardiovascular disease. Adipose tissue is a key metabolizer of testosterone to oestradiol which contributes to the testosterone-deficient state. Early studies have found that testosterone replacement therapy in men with type 2 diabetes has beneficial effects on glycaemic control, insulin resistance, and visceral adiposity. Hypogonadism is underdiagnosed in men with diabetes; however, symptoms of hypogonadism respond to testosterone replacement therapy in the majority of these men. Current knowledge and the need for larger clinical trials will be discussed in this chapter.

11.2 Insulin resistance

Insulin resistance is a central defect in the pathogenesis of the metabolic syndrome and type 2 diabetes. Visceral adiposity, genetic factors, and lack of exercise all contribute to the state of insulin resistance. Insulin resistance is directly involved with the development of several cardiovascular risk factors as shown in Figure 11.1. Any improvement in insulin sensitivity by inference would potentially lead to a reduction in cardiovascular risk.

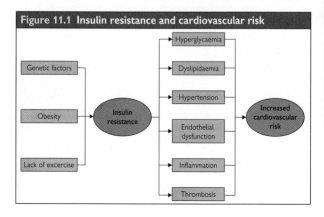

Figure 11.1 Insulin resistance and cardiovascular risk

Insulin resistance is best assessed by the euglycaemic clamp technique; however, it is time consuming. In larger studies the HOMA-IR (homeostatic model assessment of insulin resistance), an equation based on euglycaemic clamp studies, is used.

The volume of visceral fat is directly proportional to the degree of insulin resistance; however, no such relationship exists with subcutaneous fat. Blood from visceral fat drains directly to the liver via the portal vein. The liver is exposed to high concentrations of free fatty acids that decrease hepatic insulin binding, increase gluconeogenesis, and produce a deterioration in insulin resistance. The adipocytokines, interleukin (IL)-6 and tumour necrosis factor (TNF)-α, increase insulin resistance.

11.3 Epidemiological studies

11.3.1 Obesity

Obesity is associated with lower levels of total, bioavailable, and free testosterone, and sex hormone-binding globulin (SHBG). Several studies have demonstrated an inverse correlation of free and total testosterone levels with the degree of visceral fat as assessed by waist circumference and CT scanning. Testosterone–oestradiol ratios are reduced in men with obesity suggesting that the lower levels of testosterone are as a result of increased aromatase activity metabolizing testosterone to oestradiol. SHBG levels are also lower in obesity, although this does not apply to all men with this condition.

The HERITAGE (HEalth Risk factors exercise Training And Genetics) Family Study found that not all men with obesity have hypogonadism. However, hypogonadism *per se* was associated with an increased percentage of body fat, which is predominantly subcutaneous fat, but lower testosterone levels were also strongly associated with visceral adiposity. A 7.5-year follow-up study of 110 men, assessed by CT scanning, found that baseline testosterone inversely correlated with the accumulation of visceral fat but not with any other fat depots.

11.3.2 Metabolic syndrome

The metabolic syndrome comprises a cluster of cardiovascular risk factors that strongly predict the subsequent development of cardiovascular disease and type 2 diabetes. There are three commonly used definitions of the metabolic syndrome: (1) WHO (World Health Organization); (2) IDF (International Diabetes Federation); and (3) NCEP III (National Cholesterol Education Program Expert Panel III). The individual components are common to all three definitions but the emphasis and cut-off values of each differ. The components consist of visceral obesity as defined by waist circumference, glucose intolerance, hypertension, hypertriglyceridaemia, and low high-density lipoprotein-cholesterol. The different definitions are described in more detail in Table 11.1. It is important to recognize that waist circumference is affected by subcutaneous as well as visceral fat. However, waist circumference does correlate with visceral fat volumes assessed by CT, MRI, or DEXA scanning. The IDF is the most widely used where visceral obesity is an essential component of the syndrome.

Three large studies have reported that the metabolic syndrome is associated with low levels of free and total testosterone. SHBG levels are also generally lower in men with the metabolic syndrome. An increasing number of the components of the metabolic syndrome are negatively correlated with testosterone levels and associated with a higher risk of clinically relevant hypogonadism. The Quebec Family Study demonstrated that men with higher testosterone levels had a reduced risk of developing the metabolic syndrome, which was independent of age. These studies provide evidence that low testosterone levels may contribute to the development of the metabolic syndrome in men.

Table 11.1 Definition of the metabolic syndrome

	WHO	IDF	NCEP III
Essential feature	Diabetes, impaired glucose tolerance or insulin resistance[a]	Central obesity (men >94 cm waist, women >80 cm waist)	No essential feature
Diagnosis requires	Essential feature plus 2 from:	Essential feature plus 2 from:	Diagnosis requires three factors from:
	Hypertension (>140/90)	Hypertension (>130/85)	Hypertension (>130/85)
	Hypertriglyceridaemia (>1.7 mmol/l)	Hypertriglyceridaemia (>1.7 mmol/l)	Hypertriglyceridaemia (>1.7 mmol/l)
	Low HDL cholesterol[b]	Low HDL cholesterol (<1.03 mmol/l)	Low HDL cholesterol (<1.03 mmol/l)
	Central obesity[c]	Raised fasting glucose (>5.6 mmol/l)	Raised fasting glucose (>5.6 mmol/l)
	Microalbuminuria[d]		Central obesity[e]

WHO, World Health Organization; IDF, International Diabetes Federation; NCEP, National Cholesterol Education Program Expert Panel III; HDL, high-density lipoprotein. Values given are for Europids.

[a] Impaired glucose tolerance = glucose > 7.8 mmol on 2 hour glucose tolerance test. Insulin resistance = in highest quartile of relevant population.

[b] HDL cholesterol < 0.9 mmol/l in men.

[c] Waist-hip ratio > 0.9 in men or BMI greater than 30.

[d] Albumin – creatinine ratio > 30.

[e] Waist circumference > 102 cm in men.

11.3.3 **Type 2 diabetes**

Over the last 30 years cross-sectional studies have consistently demonstrated that men with type 2 diabetes have a high prevalence of low testosterone levels. There has, however, been the general perception that this is wholly due to the presence of low SHBG levels. Low SHBG levels are found in some but not all subjects with states of insulin resistance. However, some studies have found that measured free and bioavailable testosterone levels, which are independent of the SHBG level are also low. Importantly, a study published by Dhindsa and colleagues in 2004 found that approximately one-third of diabetic men have a free testosterone level (assayed by equilibrium dialysis) below the normal range. A meta-analysis of studies involving 2500 men did not find any significant difference in SHBG levels between controls and men with diabetes. Women with diabetes, however, do have lower levels of SHBG compared with those without.

Until recently, no study had assessed the prevalence of hypo-gonadism, i.e. the presence of symptoms and biochemical testosterone deficiency in a population of men with diabetes. The Barnsley Study in the UK found a high prevalence of hypogonadism with 17% of men having a total testosterone <8 nmol/l and 14% a bioavailable testosterone <2.5 nmol/l (below the normal range for each). A further 25% of men had a total testosterone between 8–12 nmol/l, while 42% had a calculated free testosterone below the normal range of 0.255nmol/l (Figure 11.2).

The prevalence of hypogonadism increased with age. SHBG levels varied below, above, and throughout the normal range. There was an inverse correlation between waist circumference and bioavailable testosterone levels. When individual symptoms of hypogonadism were analysed there was no statistical difference in patients with a total testosterone <12 nmol/l and >12 nmol/l. However, the ADAM score, taken as a cluster of three or more hypogonadal symptoms, was significantly more likely to be positive below 12 nmol/l.

11.4 **Low testosterone: a risk factor for metabolic syndrome and diabetes**

Large studies have reported that a low free or bioavailable testosterone level is an independent risk factor for the later development of the metabolic syndrome and type 2 diabetes. These studies include the MMAS (Massachusetts Male Aging Study), MRFIT (Multiple Risk Factor Intervention Trial), NHANES III (Third National Health and Nutrition Survey), and the Rancho-Bernardo Study. Two of these studies (MMAS, MRFIT) have importantly found that a low free testosterone specifically in non-obese men is an independent risk factor for

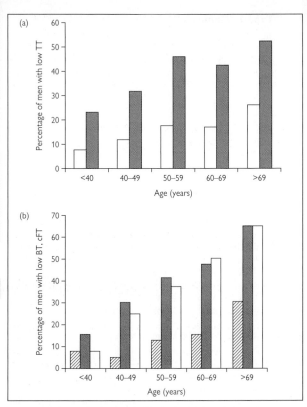

Figure 11.2 Prevalence of hypogonadism in men with type 2 diabetes (The Barnsley Study). The figures show the percentage of men with a positive symptom score and biochemical evidence of low total testosterone (a: white TT < 8 nmol/l. blue TT < 12 nmol/l) or bioactive testosterone. (b: hatched BT < 2.5 nmol/l, blue BT < 4 nmol/l, white cFT < 0.255 nmol/l).

(TT = total testosterone, BT = bioavailable testosterone, cFT = free testosterone).

Figure 11.2. Copyright © 2007. American Diabetes Association from Diabetes Care®, Vol. **30**, 2007; 911–17. Reprinted with permission from the *American Diabetes Association*.

the future development of the metabolic syndrome. The NHANES III study showed that men in the lowest compared with the highest tertile of free or bioavailable testosterone were four times more likely to have type 2 diabetes after the data was adjusted for obesity, age, and ethnicity. All studies also found that a low SHBG is an independent risk factor for the metabolic syndrome and diabetes. An 11-year follow-up study found that men with the metabolic syndrome have an increased risk of developing hypogonadism.

Furthermore, men with Klinefelter's Syndrome have a higher prevalence of diabetes. Kennedy's Syndrome (described in Chapter 2), which is due to an insensitive androgen receptor, is invariably associated with diabetes. The range of CAG repeats in a diabetic cohort was, however, similar to a healthy population. In addition, androgen suppression in men with prostate carcinoma leads to increased hazard-risk ratio for the development of diabetes.

11.5 The Hypogonadal–Obesity–Adipocytokine Cycle Hypothesis

11.5.1 The Hypogonadal–Obesity Cycle

In 1999, Cohen put forward a hypothesis to explain the relationship between obesity and increased testosterone breakdown. Aromatase activity is high in adipose tissue and is greater in visceral than subcutaneous fat. Therefore, the greater the volume of fat the more testosterone is metabolized to oestradiol. Adipocytes express androgen receptors, the density of which is positively regulated by testosterone. Testosterone inhibits the adipocyte enzyme, lipoprotein lipase, which converts free fatty acids to triglycerides and promotes their uptake into the fat cell. Lower levels of testosterone thus increase triglyceride uptake into adipocytes. Increased triglyceride uptake stimulates the conversion of pre-adipocytes into mature cells.

Higher testosterone levels stimulate pluripotent stem cells to develop into muscle cells, whereas testosterone deficiency promotes their development down the adipocyte lineage. This leads to a further increase in adipose tissue volume and hence greater overall aromatase activity, which drives the cycle forward causing further testosterone metabolism to oestradiol (see Figure 11.3).

11.5.2 The Hypogonadal–Obesity–Adipocytokine Cycle Hypothesis

The normal homeostatic response to low circulating levels of testosterone is an increased stimulation of the hypothalamic–pituitary production of luteinizing hormone (LH). The majority of men with hypogonadism, visceral obesity, and diabetes have low testosterone levels associated with normal or low levels of LH. This demonstrates a failure of the normal response. The reason for this is likely to be a combination of factors, which include the effects of oestradiol and adipocytokines. The hypogonadal–obesity–adipocytokine cycle hypothesis explains the reasons behind the failure of the body to respond to the testosterone-deficient state caused by obesity (see Figure 11.3).

There are at least five mechanisms inhibiting the hypothalamic–pituitary–testicular axis response to the state of testosterone deficiency.

- Oestradiol produced as a consequence of enhanced testosterone metabolism by aromatase inhibits LH secretion from the hypothalamic–pituitary axis. This effect has been demonstrated by the inhibitory effect of clomifene, an anti-oestrogen which inhibits the action of oestradiol on the hypothalamic–pituitary axis, increasing LH secretion.
- The proinflammatory adipocytokines IL-6 and TNFα are known to suppress the hypothalamic–pituitary axis. The higher volume of fat results in enhanced release of the adipocytokines into the circulation.
- Human obesity is associated with hypothalamic leptin resistance. The normal physiological effect of leptin is to stimulate LH release. Circulating leptin levels are directly proportional to the volume of body fat. If leptin resistance exists then the hormone fails to stimulate the hypothalamic–pituitary axis.

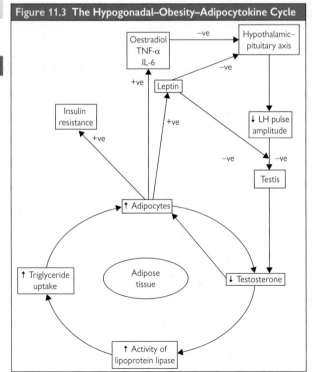

Figure 11.3 The Hypogonadal–Obesity–Adipocytokine Cycle

- Leptin also has a direct inhibitory effect on the testosterone releasing action of LH on the testis.
- There is a higher prevalence of reduced androgen receptor sensitivity (CAG repeat polymorphism) in men with obesity.

All of these factors and possibly more combine to impair the hypothalamic–pituitary–testicular axis, resulting in these men eventually becoming hypogonadal.

11.6 Diagnosis of hypogonadism

As described in Chapter 3, special attention and caution must be applied by the clinician in the diagnosis of hypogonadism in men with obesity, the metabolic syndrome, and diabetes. Specifically, the effects of obesity, age, and statin therapy on SHBG will influence the level of total testosterone. If total testosterone is <12 nmol/l in the presence of symptoms measurement should be repeated along with SHBG levels. The total testosterone and SHBG levels can then be used to calculate the free and/or bioavailable testosterone. If the total testosterone is <8 nmol/l then there is little doubt that the patient is hypogonadal. Between 8 and 12 nmol/l if the free testosterone is <0.255 pmol/l or bioavailable testosterone <2.5 nmol/l (depending on local laboratory validation and normal ranges) in the presence of symptoms, this would support a diagnosis of hypogonadism. If the free testosterone and bioavailable testosterone are low-normal and clinical suspicion of hypogonadism is high, a trial of testosterone replacement therapy for 3 months could be considered. The diagnosis of hypogonadism can be difficult to assess. The decisions to investigate an underlying cause and to treat should be made by an experienced clinician.

11.6.1 Gonadotrophins

The Barnsley study found that 74% of men with hypogonadism had either low or normal gonadotrophin levels. Of these, 64% had LH levels within the normal range. The probable explanation for this is described above in the section on the Hypogonadal–Obesity–Adipocytokine Cycle hypothesis, which would be consistent with hypogonadotrophic hypogonadism. This was also found in the Dhindsa study discussed above. The remaining 26% had elevated levels consistent with primary gonadal failure which included men with previously undiagnosed Klinefelter's Syndrome.

11.7 Testosterone and insulin sensitivity

11.7.1 Healthy populations

The San Antonio Heart Study (1994) found that free testosterone levels correlated inversely with glucose and insulin levels. The French

Telecom study (1992) of 1292 healthy non-diabetic men also demonstrated that total testosterone levels correlated negatively with serum insulin. Furthermore, a population study from Finland found that free and total testosterone inversely correlated with insulin resistance.

11.7.2 **Hypogonadism**

Insulin sensitivity is reduced in men with hypogonadism. There is an inverse relationship between total testosterone and insulin resistance. Androgen suppression in healthy men using gonadotrophin-releasing hormone agonists, anti-androgens, or a combination of both results in an increase in insulin levels but has no significant effect on fasting blood glucose. However, treatment of prostate carcinoma with gonadotrophin-releasing hormone agonists produces insulin resistance, hyperglycaemia, and an increased risk of developing diabetes. A follow-up study of 73,196 men with loco-regional prostate carcinoma, of which one-third were treated with gonadotrophin-releasing hormone agonists, found a significantly increased hazard ratio of 1.44 for incident diabetes. Surgical castration also increases fasting and postprandial glucose and insulin levels. In addition, androgen suppression for prostate cancer therapy in men with diabetes results in deterioration of glycaemic control. Testosterone substitution in hypogonadal men improves insulin sensitivity.

11.7.3 **Obesity**

Several studies have shown that testosterone substitution therapy improves insulin resistance in obese men. These improvements correlated with a reduction in central obesity. It is important to note however that supraphysiological testosterone levels lead to a reduction in insulin sensitivity.

11.7.4 **Mechanisms**

There are several potential mechanisms by which testosterone improves insulin sensitivity. The study described above demonstrates that testosterone reduces visceral mass, which by inference would improve insulin resistance.

Mitochondrial function as assessed by maximal aerobic capacity on exercise testing and the expression of ubiquinol cytochrome c reductase-binding (UQCRB) protein gene in muscle, is impaired in men with type 2 diabetes.

There are also *in vitro* data that testosterone stimulates the release of insulin from isolated pancreatic β cells. This effect was of rapid onset, which implies that this action is mediated via a non-genomic effect.

11.8 **Type 2 diabetes: testosterone replacement therapy**

A pilot (double blind placebo-controlled crossover) study of 7 months duration in men with type 2 diabetes and hypogonadism has shown that testosterone replacement therapy improves insulin resistance (as measured by Homeostatic Model for Assessment of Insulin Resistance (HOMA-IR), fasting blood glucose, and HbA1c (mean: 0.37% over 3 months). In addition, it resulted in a reduced waist circumference, and a lowering of leptin and cholesterol levels. This study also demonstrated a significant benefit of testosterone compared with placebo in reducing hypogonadal symptoms. Two other studies (non-placebo-controlled) with testosterone have also demonstrated an improvement in HbA1c. The beneficial effect on HbA1c may potentially in the longer-term improve as it can take up to 18 months to achieve the maximal effect of testosterone replacement on body composition. Furthermore thiazolidenedione insulin sensitizers used in current practice require four to six months to achieve their maximal effect. No studies on testosterone substitution in the metabolic syndrome have yet been published. Larger studies in metabolic syndrome and diabetes are underway.

No studies on testosterone substitution in the metabolic syndrome have yet been published.

However just prior to publication of this book such a study was presented at the Endocrine Society meeting in San Francisco, ENDO 08.

The TIMES2 (Testosterone replacement In hypogonadal men with either MEtabolic Syndrome or type 2 diabetes) Study is a multi-centre European double-blind, placebo-controlled study over a 12 month treatment period involving 220 subjects. Subjects were treated with a metered-dose of 2% testosterone gel with dose titration to achieve a serum total testosterone of >17 nmol/l. The primary outcome studied was the effect of testosterone on insulin resistance as assessed by HOMA-IR. The preliminary analysis of the results has shown a significant improvement in insulin resistance in men with type 2 diabetes with a trend to reduction in insulin resistance, which approached significance in the men with metabolic syndrome without diabetes. The study also demonstrated a significant benefit on the IIEF (International Index of Erectile Function) score. Secondary outcome analyses on effects on glycaemic control, waist circumference and other cardiovascular risk factors are awaited.

According to the UKPDS (United Kingdom Prospective Diabetes Study), an improvement in the HbA1c of 1% leads to a: (1) 21% reduction in diabetes-related death; (2) 16% reduction in myocardial infarction; (3) 43% reduction in peripheral vascular disease; and (4) 37% reduction in microvascular complications. Therefore any reduction in HbA1c can be translated into a beneficial effect on clinical outcomes. Longer-term studies are required to determine if this beneficial effect of testosterone is maintained or even enhances over subsequent months, as the positive effects on body composition may continue to improve for up to 18–24 months.

11.9 Cardiovascular risk factors

The association of testosterone with cardiovascular risk factors, which are also common to the metabolic syndrome and diabetes, are dealt with in Chapter 12.

11.10 Erectile dysfunction

Erectile dysfunction is a common complication of diabetes with reports of up to 70% of diabetic men being affected. The main cause of the erectile dysfunction is vascular disease; however, hypogonadism, neuropathy, and drug side-effects can be involved in varying degrees. The severity of the erectile dysfunction is inversely correlated with the bioavailable and free testosterone. Erectile dysfunction may be the first presentation of diabetes or cardiovascular disease. The diameter of the penile artery is approximately half that of the coronary artery and hence more likely to be affected earlier. Erectile dysfunction is the herald of future cardiovascular events.

11.11 Conclusions

There is now a large body of evidence that there is a high prevalence of hypogonadism in men with the metabolic syndrome and type 2 diabetes. The diagnosis of hypogonadism and treatment with testosterone substitution to achieve circulating levels within the physiological range can lead to improvement and, in many, resolution of symptoms attributable to testosterone deficiency. Early reports, albeit short-term studies with small numbers, have demonstrated beneficial effects of testosterone replacement therapy on insulin resistance, glycaemic control, waist circumference, and other cardiovascular risk factors. There is a clear need for larger and longer-term studies to determine if these effects persist. Until then testosterone cannot be indicated for the treatment of diabetes; however, testosterone is a recognized and established treatment for hypogonadism.

Key references

Dhindsa S, Prabhakar S, Sethi M, Bandyopadhyay A, Chaudhuri A, Dandona P. (2004). Frequent occurrence of hypogonadotrophic hypogonadism in type 2 diabetes. *J Clin Endocrinol Metab* **89**: 5462–8.

Ding EL, Song Y, Malik VS, Liu S. (2006). Sex differences of endogenous sex hormones and risk of type 2 diabetes. *JAMA* **295**: 1288–99.

Jones TH. (2007). Testosterone associations with erectile dysfunction, diabetes and the metabolic syndrome. *Eur Urol* **6 (Suppl)**: 847–57.

Kapoor D, Malkin CJ, Channer KS, Jones TH. (2005). Androgens insulin resistance and vascular disease in men. *Clin Endocrinol* **63**: 239–50.

Kapoor D, Goodwin E, Channer KS, Jones TH. (2006). Testosterone replacement therapy improves insulin resistance, glycaemic control, visceral adiposity. *Eur J Endocrinol* **154**: 899–906.

Kapoor D, Aldred H, Channer KS, Jones TH. (2007). Clinical and biochemical assessment of hypogonadism in men with type 2 diabetes: correlations with bioavailable testosterone and visceral adiposity. *Diabetes Care* **30**: 911–17.

Keating NL, O'Malley AJ, Smith MR. (2006). Diabetes and cardiovascular disease during androgen deprivation therapy for prostate cancer. *J Clin Oncol* **24**: 4448–56.

Chapter 12

The heart and cardiovascular disease

T. Hugh Jones

> **Key points**
> - Male gender is a major cardiovascular risk factor that has not been adequately explained.
> - Low testosterone levels are associated with the presence and the degree of atherosclerosis.
> - Low testosterone levels are associated with several cardiovascular risk factors that include visceral obesity, insulin resistance, dyslipidaemia, and hypertension.
> - Testosterone therapy improves exercise-induced cardiac ischaemia in men with chronic stable angina.
> - Testosterone therapy improves functional exercise capacity in men with moderate chronic heart failure.

12.1 Introduction

Cardiovascular disease is the most common cause of death in the Western world. Men are two to three times more likely to die from coronary heart disease (CHD) than women even after controlling for sex differences in smoking, obesity, and other factors. This ratio is present in all Western countries independent of different rates of overall CHD mortality.

The aetiology of CHD is multifactorial and the relative weighting of each cardiovascular risk factor will vary between individuals and sexes. Male gender is an important risk factor that has been relatively ignored in the medical community as it has been felt that little can be done to change its influence.

There has been a premise that testosterone is 'bad for the heart', but there is little to no evidence to support this hypothesis. There are three pieces of evidence that are based on tenuous extrapolations:

1. Oestrogens in women may have a protective effect against atherosclerosis based on the low prevalence of CHD prior to the menopause. Commentators have suggested that low oestrogen levels in men leads to the loss of this atheroprotective mechanism.

2. There are a few case reports of men using anabolic steroids who present with myocardial infarction. They are used in very high androgen doses resulting in markedly elevated supraphysi-ological levels of androgens when compared to natural testos-terone (up to 100–1000 fold higher). Anabolic steroids are mainly non-aromatizable. There are no prospective or retrospective studies in this group.

3. Clinically induced hypogonadism in young men in some studies leads to a lowering of high-density lipoprotein (HDL) cholesterol. This does not, however, occur in older men and there is some recent evidence that in the longer term HDL cholesterol rises with testosterone substitution.

12.2 Epidemiological studies

12.2.1 Mortality studies

There is accumulating evidence that CHD and related mortality are associated with low testosterone levels. Two studies, one of men who had previously been hospitalized (Veterans Study) and the other of men in an ageing community dwelling population (the Rancho-Bernardo Study), had a significantly reduced survival time if the baseline testosterone was less than 8 mmol/l compared with a level >12 mmol/l. Furthermore, both studies found an excess incidence of cardiovascular mortality. The European Prospective Investigation Into Cancer in Norfolk (EPIC-Norfolk) study (n = 11,606 men) found an increase in mortality due to cardiovascular disease with lowest quartile of testosterone. However, the Massachusetts Male Aging Study (MMAS), which at the outset was studying a younger more healthy population, found only a weak association of increased mortality in men with lower testosterone levels but no association with CHD. The Rancho-Bernardo Study and the MMAS both found that low testosterone status is associated with an increased risk of mortality from respiratory disease.

12.2.2 Androgen suppression

A large study of 73,196 men with loco-regional prostate carcinoma, of which approximately one-third were treated with testosterone suppression (gonadotrophin-releasing hormone (GnRH) analogue therapy), found that over a 7-year follow-up period the hazard ratio was significantly increased for ischaemic heart disease, myocardial infarction, diabetes, and cardiovascular death.

12.2.3 **Coronary heart disease**

Several cross-sectional studies have been reported, of which half showed no association of CHD end-points and the other half found a significant association with low testosterone levels. Interestingly, the studies that demonstrated this relationship measured or calculated either free or bioavailable testosterone. One study compared testosterone levels in men with significant CHD (>75% stenosis of at least one coronary artery at angiography) with a control group of men with normal coronary angiograms. This study reported that both measured bioavailable and calculated free testosterone levels were lower in the CHD group. Total testosterone approached, but did not attain, significance.

12.2.4 **Carotid and aortic atherosclerosis**

Four studies have all reported that the carotid intimal media thickness is negatively correlated with testosterone. One study that was followed up after 4 years found that men in the lowest tertile of either total or free testosterone levels had the greatest progression of intimal media thickness. The Rotterdam Study of elderly men demonstrated that aortic atheroma, as assessed by the degree of aortic calcification on X-ray, was again inversely proportional to testosterone levels.

12.3 **Cardiovascular risk factors**

The major cardiovascular risk factors are family history of CHD, smoking, visceral obesity, diabetes, the metabolic syndrome, hypertension, dyslipidaemia, lack of exercise and fruit and vegetables in the diet, and male gender. In addition, a pro-coaguable and pro-inflammatory milieu are contributory factors. The associations of testosterone deficiency with these risk factors are discussed below.

12.3.1 **Visceral obesity**

Visceral obesity as demonstrated by the INTERHEART Study is an important modifiable factor for risk of first myocardial infarction. As discussed in Chapter 11, visceral obesity is a key cause of insulin resistance and, therefore, atherosclerosis. There is a higher incidence of testosterone deficiency in men with visceral obesity and related disorders. The hypogonadal–obesity–adipocytokine cycle produces a state where testosterone is rapidly metabolized and the hypothalamic–pituitary axis is impaired and unable to respond and hence replenish testosterone levels.

12.3.2 **Glucose intolerance and diabetes**

Diabetes and the metabolic syndrome are major cardiovascular risk factors. As described in Chapter 11 testosterone deficiency has a higher prevalence in these conditions and is associated with insulin resistance.

12.3.3 **Dyslipidaemia**

Testosterone deficiency is associated with changes in the lipid profile, which are consistent with a pro-atherogenic milieu. The majority of cross-sectional studies have found that testosterone has a negative correlation with total cholesterol, low-density lipoprotein (LDL) cholesterol, and triglycerides. Some studies, however, have not confirmed these associations. Healthy and diabetic men have a significant positive correlation between testosterone and HDL cholesterol levels.

The effects of testosterone replacement therapy on lipid levels are also conflicting. In healthy young men where hypogonadism was chemically induced, testosterone replacement therapy produced a rise in total and LDL cholesterol and a fall in HDL cholesterol. Yet in older men, testosterone substitution reduces total and LDL cholesterol with no change in HDL cholesterol. A meta-analysis of several studies has demonstrated that testosterone replacement produces a reduction in total and LDL cholesterol and a small decrease in HDL cholesterol. It is, however, important to note that the effects of testosterone substitution are likely to be dependent on the duration of treatment as observed with statin therapy, and other factors such as age. In the short term, testosterone may enhance shuttling of the cholesterol to the liver, resulting in consumption of HDL cholesterol and in the longer term there may be stabilization.

Interestingly, two studies have reported that testosterone therapy in men already receiving statin treatment for over 1 and 3 months generates a further small fall in total cholesterol. Longer-term, in particular cardiovascular outcome studies, will be required to establish any benefits on the lipid profile and reduction in cardiovascular events.

12.3.4 **Coagulation**

Several studies have demonstrated that testosterone deficiency is associated with a pro-coaguable state. Major clotting factors, that have been shown to be linked to testosterone levels are: fibrinogen, plasminogen-activator inhibitor type 1 (PAI-1), and tissue plasminogen activator (tPA). In cross-sectional studies low testosterone levels are associated with higher fibrinogen concentrations. Testosterone replacement has in one study been reported to lower fibrinogen levels, although others have not detected a significant change.

Serum tPA was positively correlated with testosterone levels, while PAI-1 was negatively correlated. Factor VII, which is involved in the conversion of prothrombin to thrombin, correlates inversely with testosterone. Myocardial infarction is associated with a fall in tPA and rise in PAI-1 levels. These changes are accompanied by a fall in testosterone. Whether or not these are coincidental or causally related is not apparent. However, it has been demonstrated that testosterone replacement therapy in hypogonadal men and dehydroepiandrosterone treatment in normal men causes a lowering of elevated PAI-1 levels. Testosterone administration in men with chronic stable angina, which included eugonadal as well as hypogonadal men, showed no change in tPA, PAI-1, or fibrinogen.

One of the complications of testosterone treatment is a raised haematocrit caused by increased erythropoiesis. Polycythaemia is associated with hyperviscosity and therefore an increased risk of thrombosis. Monitoring of the haematocrit is essential to the management of testosterone therapy and the dose can be lowered to reduce these changes. A slight elevation of the haematocrit is unlikely to be associated with an increased risk; however, each patient and their co-morbid state needs to be assessed on an individual basis.

In recent years there have been concerns regarding the increased risk of thrombo-embolism with hormone replacement therapy in women. The evidence in men suggests that this is not the case with testosterone replacement therapy and indeed there may be a beneficial effect in hypogonadal subjects.

12.3.5 Hypertension

Case-controlled studies show that men with hypertension have lower testosterone levels than men with normal blood pressure. A similar relationship has been observed in treated or untreated men with hypertension and normotensive men who have CHD. Testosterone therapy has in only one study lowered diastolic blood pressure by 5 mmHg, whereas other studies have not demonstrated any significant change. Potentially, testosterone may lower blood pressure by reducing peripheral vascular resistance. There also may be an effect of testosterone on activation of the renin–angiotensin system.

12.3.6 Endothelial dysfunction

The data on the effects of testosterone on endothelial dysfunction assessed by flow-mediated vasodilation of the brachial artery are conflicting. Further research in this area is needed to clarify whether or not testosterone has beneficial or adverse effects on endothelial dysfunction. (see Section 12.6 for more detail).

12.3.7 Testosterone and inflammation

Atherosclerosis is intimately linked with a pro-inflammatory milieu. A local inflammatory response is integral to the early stages of the pathogenesis and is also involved in the instability of the established plaque. Inflammatory proteins, which include C-reactive protein, fibrinogen, interleukin (IL)-1, and IL-6, can be elevated in the circulation of people with atherosclerosis. Little is known regarding the role of testosterone on the immune system. Isolated case reports have described beneficial effects of testosterone therapy, for example, there is an association between systemic lupus erythematosus and Klinefelter's Syndrome. Testosterone substitution to treat hypogonadism has resulted in an improvement in the systemic lupus erythematosus.

Serum IL-1β levels increase with atherosclerotic burden in men with CHD. Furthermore, the elevation of IL-1β was higher in the hypogonadal group. It is not clear, however, whether or not this is a cause or effect situation or a combination of actions. Serum levels of IL-6 and C-reactive protein correlate inversely with testosterone in hypogonadal men with type 2 diabetes. Testosterone replacement therapy in a group of hypogonadal men, which included a significant proportion of men with CHD, lowered circulating levels of tumour necrosis factor-α (TNF-α) and IL-1β and increased levels of the anti-inflammatory and atheroprotective cytokine IL-10. Also, young males presenting with delayed puberty as a result of idiopathic hypogonadism have higher serum levels of inflammatory cytokines than normal controls. Conversely, GnRH-induced hypogonadism in elderly normal men increases serum IL-6 and TNF-α levels. A longer-term effect of GnRH analogue therapy in this study was not undertaken. Soluble IL-6 receptor, which has pro-inflammatory effects, also inversely correlates with testosterone but there was no association with IL-6, IL-1β, TNFα, or C-reactive protein.

In vitro studies have provided some evidence that testosterone suppresses pro-inflammatory cytokines and stimulates anti-inflammatory cytokines from leucocytes. The castration of mice also produces a rise in endogenous TNF-α levels. A recent study by Corrales and co-workers has demonstrated that androgen replacement therapy in men with type 2 diabetes suppresses *ex-vivo* IL-1β, IL-6, and TNF-α secretion from antigen-presenting cells. However, lipopolysaccharide or interferon-γ stimulation of these cells showed no differences in cytokine release before and after treatment.

The effects of testosterone on adhesion molecule expression are less clear. Testosterone reduces TNF-α-stimulated VCAM-1 (vascular adhesion molecule type 1) expression in human aortic endothelial cells and in female origin human umbilical vein endothelial cells (HUVECs). Dihydrotestosterone enhances monocyte adhesion to IL-1β-stimulated HUVECs and human umbilical artery endothelial cells from male origin, and increases IL-1β-induced VCAM-1 expression in these cells, via activation of nuclear factor-κB.

Overall the evidence suggests that testosterone has an anti-inflammatory effect.

12.4 **Testosterone and atherosclerosis**

There are no human studies that have been performed to determine whether or not testosterone therapy improves or slows down the progression of atherosclerosis. However, as described above, men in the lower tertile of testosterone levels have a greater progression of intimal media thickness than those in the upper tertile. There are, however, a few reports from animal work that demonstrate testosterone prevents, and can reverse or ameliorate, early athero-genesis. Orchidectomized male rabbits fed a pro-atherogenic diet develop cholesterol accumulation in the aorta. This cholesterol deposition was significantly reduced in a similar group treated with testosterone supplementation. These effects appear to be gender-specific with oestrogen having no protective effect in male rabbits. A further study has demonstrated that testosterone replacement in mature castrated rabbits again prevented atherosclerosis. In untreated rabbits there was a doubling of the degree of lipid deposition, which was ameliorated by treatment with testosterone.

Physiological testosterone substitution also reduces the development of early atherosclerosis in orchidectomized LDL receptor knockout mice, which were given a cholesterol-enriched diet. Interestingly, when anastrozole (an aromatase inhibitor) was given along with the testosterone, the atheroprotective effect was blocked. This suggests that oestrogen may be involved in the protective role.

The testicular feminized mouse (tfm) has a frameshift mutation in the classic androgen receptor, which results in complete inactivity of the receptor. This mutation is associated with low circulating testo-sterone levels as a result of 17α-hydroxylase deficiency. Tfm mice fed with high cholesterol leads to weight gain and the formation of lipid streaks within the aortic root, whereas no lipid deposition is observed in the wild-type littermate control. Physiological testosterone replacement in the tfm mouse protects against lipid deposition and the early development of atherogenesis. This work shows that the androgen receptor plays an important part in protection against lipid deposition during the early stage of atherogenesis in this model. Co-treatment with either anastrozole or an oestradiol β-receptor antagonist partially inhibited the beneficial effect of testosterone. These data demonstrate in an animal model that testosterone has an atheroprotective action, which is mediated through mechanisms independent of the classical androgen receptor. The evidence suggests that this effect is mediated in part through oestradiol and part by a direct effect of testosterone *per se*.

12.5 **Testosterone and angina**

Testosterone was first used as a treatment for angina in both men and women in the early 1940s. Several case reports proclaimed that the administration of testosterone propionate improved the symptoms and frequency of angina in the majority of patients. A placebo-controlled study in 1977 found that testosterone treatment in 50 men with CHD produced a 32% reduction in time to 1 mm ST-segment depression on exercise treadmill testing (the gold standard test to assess cardiac ischaemia) after 1 month and 51% after 3 months. Oral testosterone treatment in a cohort of 62 elderly Chinese men with angina in a 1-month placebo crossover study led to improvements in ischaemia and anginal symptoms. A double-blind, randomized placebo-controlled, add-on trial using transdermal testosterone patches (5 mg/day for 3 months) in a group of men with chronic stable angina, who were unselected for baseline hypogonadism, showed that testosterone induced a significant benefit on time to 1 mm ST-segment depression by 37% (52 seconds). Many of these men were already treated with two or three anti-anginal drugs and, pharmacologically, an increase of 52 seconds is greater than that which would be expected for the addition of a third or fourth drug. The study also showed that the lower the baseline bioavailable testosterone, the greater the beneficial effect of testosterone therapy on the time to ischaemia. A further study involving men with angina and overt hypogonadism (mean testosterone approximately 4 nmol/l [normal range 8.3–30]) reported that 1 month's treatment with testosterone led to a 74 seconds improvement in time to 1 mm ST depression.

Acute administration of testosterone directly into the coronary circulation at cardiac catheterization in humans leads to a rapid vasodilatation and an increase in coronary blood flow within 2–3 min of treatment. This effect is dose-dependent and occurs at testosterone concentrations within the normal physiological range. Furthermore an acute intravenous bolus of testosterone prior to exercise treadmill testing results in a significant improvement in ischaemia. In these studies, the resulting serum testosterone levels were well above the physiological range. The mechanism mediating the rapid onset of action is non-genomic and is likely to be via an action on calcium and potassium voltage-operated channels as described below. The mechanism(s) that explain the sustained action of testosterone on cardiac ischaemia are not known, although an effect of testosterone on vessel tone would again be likely.

12.6 **Testosterone as a vasodilator**

The majority of studies using isolated blood vessels *in vitro* have shown that testosterone acts as a vasodilator. Animal studies have shown that testosterone stimulates vasodilatation in different vascular beds, which include rabbit coronary arteries and aorta, mouse iliac arteries, rat coronary, mesenteric and pulmonary arteries. Similar effects of testosterone have been demonstrated in isolated human vessels comprising mesenteric and pulmonary arteries and, more recently, gluteal arteries from subcutaneous skin. After 3 months of androgen suppression treatment for prostate cancer, vascular stiffness (measured using pulse-wave analysis) increased in the radial artery and the aorta.

The vasodilatory effect is of rapid-onset, acting within 2–3 min of testosterone administration. The speed of action, and the findings that the effect is not blocked by flutamide (classic androgen receptor blocker) and persists in the testicular feminized mouse (which has an inactive androgen receptor) strongly suggest that it is independent of the classical androgen receptor. The effect is also independent of the endothelium, nitric oxide, and cyclo-oxygenase activity. Pharmacological concentrations are required in the isolated artery model to elicit the vasodilatory effect. However, more recent studies on isolated vascular smooth muscle cells have demonstrated direct inhibitory effects on calcium channels at physiological concentrations.

The exact mechanism(s) by which testosterone mediates its vasodilatatory action, may be either through activation of potassium channels or blocking calcium channels. Testosterone has been shown to activate calcium-sensitive potassium channels and to have a calcium antagonistic action. Electrophysiological and microfluorimetry studies in a vascular smooth muscle cell line have provided evidence that at physiological concentrations testosterone inhibits L-type voltage-gated calcium channels (VGCCs). The inhibitory effect of testosterone was also rapid in this system occurring within 2 min. It was also shown that 5β-dihydrotestosterone blocked L-type calcium channels with an IC50 of 6.1 nM compared with an IC50 of 3.1 nM for testosterone. This confirms that testosterone alone is blocking these channels and is not dependent on conversion to oestradiol.

The L-type calcium channel consists of four protein subunits of which the main α1c subunit forms the pore. Human embryonic kidney cells (HEK293, which do not express calcium channels) transfected with the α1c subunit exhibited a similar inhibitory action. This implies that testosterone acts as a calcium channel blocker and has a similar action to commonly prescribed calcium channel blocking drugs, such as dihydropyridines, which include nifedipine and amlodipine routinely used for the treatment of angina and hypertension.

Testosterone therapy in men with CHD has been shown to enhance flow-mediated brachial artery vasodilatation, which occurs as a consequence of nitric oxide release from the endothelium. These changes are evident in the short and longer term. Conversely, hypogonadal men without cardiovascular disease have a higher flow and nitrate-mediated brachial artery vasodilatation. Testosterone substitution leads to a restoration of brachial artery reactivity to normal. Several other studies have shown conflicting effects of testosterone on brachial artery reactivity with studies on other vessels. For example, flow-mediated but not nitrate-mediated brachial artery vasodilatation increases in men with prostate carcinoma treated with either chemical or surgical castration. However, arterial stiffness as assessed by the augmentation index in Doppler studies in the radial artery and aorta increases after induction of hypogonadism.

12.7 **Chronic heart failure**

Chronic heart failure is a condition associated with a high morbidity and mortality equivalent to many cancers. The 1-year mortality after hospital discharge is as high as 30%. Chronic heart failure is associated with an excess of catabolic hormones and a relative deficiency of anabolic hormones. Testosterone levels have been reported to be low in this condition. Testosterone therapy has been contraindicated in men with chronic heart failure. The basis for this is not fully clear but is likely to be due to the fact that older parenteral preparations of testosterone could be associated with fluid retention. Newer preparations do not appear to have this problem. Until recently no studies of testosterone therapy have been performed in men with heart failure.

Acute administration of buccal testosterone to men with chronic heart failure showed a fall in peripheral vascular resistance and reduction in cardiac index, which is a measure of cardiac function. A small non-blinded study found that the anabolic steroid oxymethalone lowered levels of brain naturetic peptide (a substance elevated in heart failure) and reduced left ventricular mass. A pilot study over a 3-month period demonstrated that testosterone therapy using intramuscular testosterone esters (Sustanon®, 200 mg fortnightly) resulted in an improvement in symptoms and functional exercise capacity. Functional exercise capacity as assessed by the Incremental Shuttle Walk Test is a highly reproducible test, which is the strongest independent predictor of peak VO_2. A further longer-term study of 12 months has been conducted using physiological testosterone replacement therapy in the form of the testosterone transdermal patch (5 mg Andropatch®). This was a double-blind randomized placebo-controlled study of 76 men with chronic heart failure who had a mean ejection fraction of 32.5%, i.e. moderate heart failure. This study again showed a benefit of testosterone therapy with a significant improvement in functional exercise capacity and with one-third of subjects improving their New York Heart Association Class of heart failure. Testosterone-treated subjects maintained systolic blood pressure and there was an increase in left ventricular cavity length and a trend to a reduction in left ventricular mass index. There was no significant improvement in muscle strength or thigh and muscle size when assessed by CT scanning. No changes in mood were detected. The effects were maximal after 3 months and maintained for the 12-month study period. There was a positive correlation of the improvement in functional exercise capacity with a change in bioavailable testosterone from baseline. There was no increase in serious adverse events and the only death during the study period was in the placebo group. Importantly, there was only a slight but not clinically significant increase in the haematocrit.

Heart failure is a state of insulin resistance and, interestingly, testosterone therapy results in an increase in insulin sensitivity in men with moderate chronic heart failure.

In patients with chronic heart failure, similar to patients with metastatic cancer, the improvement in life expectancy may not be realistic, whereas a benefit in quality of life is! Although these studies are small they are proof of concept and should lead to larger studies in the future.

12.8 Conclusions

There is accumulating evidence that testosterone is a hormone with major vascular, metabolic, and immunological actions, in addition to the classic sex and anabolic functions. There is also increasing evidence that atherosclerosis is associated with low testosterone states. It is not clear if testosterone deficiency is a cardiovascular risk factor or a consequence of the disease. It is likely, however, from the data presented that it is a combination of the two. Studies also support the hypothesis that testosterone deficiency is associated with adverse effects on several cardiovascular risk factors. Importantly, testosterone replacement therapy can improve insulin resistance, glycaemic control in diabetics, visceral adiposity, lipid, coagulation, and inflammatory profiles to promote a less atherogenic milieu. Animal studies provide supportive evidence that testosterone therapy can ameliorate atherogenesis. There is also sufficient published data to suggest that men treated for prostate cancer with GnRH analogues or surgical orchidectomy should be treated for primary prevention of cardiovascular disease. This would include reduction in cardiovascular risk factors, surveillance for diabetes, and treatment where appropriate with aspirin and statins.

Early, albeit short-term and small, clinical trials have also demonstrated beneficial effects of testosterone therapy in angina and chronic heart failure as well as type 2 diabetes. It is important to note that data sheets from pharmaceutical companies state that testosterone replacement for hypogonadism should be used with caution in men with coexisting cardiovascular disease and is contraindicated in men with congestive cardiac failure. The rationale for its contraindication in heart failure is based on the older formulations of testosterone causing fluid retention. There is, however, no evidence that this occurs with the new formulations, provided physiological levels of testosterone replacement are achieved. There is now a significant body of evidence available to recommend that larger and longer-term studies of testosterone replacement therapy in cardiovascular disease should be performed.

Key references

English KM, Steeds RP, Jones TH, Diver MJ, Channer KS. (2000). Low-dose transdermal testosterone therapy improves angina threshold in men with chronic stable angina: a randomized, double-blind, placebo-controlled study. *Circulation* **102**: 1906–11.

Jones RD, Nettleship JE, Kapoor D, Jones TH, Channer KS. (2005). Testosterone and atherosclerosis in aging men: purported association and clinical implications. *Am J Cardiovasc Drugs* **5**: 141–54.

Jones TH, Jones RD, Channer KS. (2003). *Testosterone and cardiovascular disorders. Recent research developments in endocrinology and metabolism 1*, pp. 143–68. Transworld Research Network, Kerala, India.

Malkin CJ, Pugh PJ, West JN, van Beek EJR, Jones TH, Channer KS. (2006). Testosterone therapy in moderate severity heart failure: a double-blind randomized placebo controlled trial. *Eur Heart J* **27**: 57–64.

Wu FCW, von Eckardstein A. (2003). Androgens and coronary artery disease. *Endocr Rev* **24**: 183–217.

Chapter 13

Testosterone and the brain

Bradley D. Anawalt

Key points

- Testosterone and its metabolites positively modulate certain aspects of male cognitive function such as visuospatial, verbal, and working memory.
- Serum testosterone levels may have a U-shaped relationship with male cognitive function; higher and lower serum testosterone levels may be associated with worse function.
- In hypogonadal men, testosterone therapy improves cognitive function, mood, and libido.
- At usual dosages testosterone does not increase aggression.
- It is unknown if testosterone supplementation in ageing men with declining testosterone levels may prevent cognitive decline and dementia.

13.1 Testosterone and the male brain

Testosterone exerts important biological effects on brain development and function throughout male life. The effects of testosterone (and dihydrotestosterone) act directly on the male brain via androgen receptors, and indirectly when testosterone is aromatized to oestrogen, which then interacts with oestrogen receptors. Androgen and oestrogen receptors are widespread in the male brain, and there is evidence of local conversion of testosterone to oestradiol and dihydrotestosterone in a variety of brain loci.

The developmental effects of androgens include 'masculinization' of the male fetus leading to permanent behavioural effects and the well known increases in sexual desire during male puberty. In adult men, androgens and oestrogens modulate important cognitive functions such as visuospatial memory, verbal memory, and fluency as well as sexual desire and fantasies. In addition, sex steroid hormones may act to preserve normal neuronal function and viability in the brains of ageing men.

13.1.1 **Effects on the developing brain**

Early neural effects of androgens are often characterized as 'organizational' effects that are defined as permanent alterations in neural organization due to exposure during early development. Neural effects of androgens in adults are often described as 'activational', a term that refers to the effects of circulating sex steroids that modulate existing steroid hormone-response neuronal pathways.

Animal studies suggest that androgens probably induce differentiation of brain regions, such as the hypothalamus, hippocampus, and the regions of the cerebral cortex. These organizational effects have long-term effects on sexual behaviour, memory, and visuospatial ability. (Visuospatial ability is broadly defined as the ability to mentally apprehend the forms, shapes, and positions of visually perceived objects, and to manipulate these representations mentally.) In experimental models, male rats outperform female rats in tests of visuospatial ability. Female rats treated with androgens late in gestation perform comparably with male rats on tests of visuospatial ability, while male rats treated with the anti-androgen flutamide late in gestation and castrated at birth perform worse than control male rats and comparably with female rats.

In humans, androgens also appear to induce early organizational effects that favour visuospatial ability. Individuals with androgen insensitivity are genotypic males that appear phenotypically female despite normal male levels of circulating testosterone. Individuals with androgen insensitivity have lower than usual visuospatial brain function compared with normal controls. Conversely, girls with congenital adrenal hyperplasia, a syndrome associated with the overproduction of adrenal androgens from the prenatal period to adulthood, outperform controls on visuospatial tests.

Androgens have favourable effects on 'working memory', the ability to hold and manipulate information 'in the mind' over brief periods of time. This effect appears to be activational. For example, older men with low or low-normal testosterone levels demonstrate improvement on tests of working memory after testosterone supplementation. Likewise, in girls with Turner's syndrome, a genetic disorder associated with ovarian failure and concomitant sex steroid hormone deficiency, exogenous androgens improve working memory.

13.2 Effects on brain function in men

Although there are several epidemiological studies examining the relationship between endogenous sex hormones and cognitive function (e.g. visuospatial ability) in normal men, the results have been inconsistent and often conflicting. A popular explanation for these inconsistent epidemiological results has been that circulating endogenous testosterone levels have a U-shaped relationship with cognitive function; optimal cognitive function occurs in the window between very low and very high circulating levels.

Dose–response studies of exogenous testosterone on cognitive function in men are also inconsistent. In small studies of normal young men, high dosages of exogenous testosterone appear to have little effect on cognitive function. In older men with low-normal serum testosterone levels, high-dosage exogenous testosterone may adversely affect cognitive function.

13.2.1 Cognitive effects in hypogonadism

Small studies have shown that hypogonadal men have lower visuospatial ability compared with eugonadal men. Testosterone administration to hypogonadal men increases these abilities. These effects of testosterone administration are associated with increased blood flow to the midbrain and frontal gyrus and increased activity in several regions of the cerebral cortex. Other studies and clinical observation suggest that restoration of normal circulating testosterone levels improves verbal memory, speed of informational responsiveness, and concentration in hypogonadal men. One small study has suggested that the positive effects of androgen therapy on verbal memory in hypogonadal men are mediated via aromatization to oestrogen, whereas the positive effects on spatial memory are mediated directly via the androgen receptor.

13.2.2 Behavioural effects in hypogonadism

Studies have consistently demonstrated that exogenous testosterone increases sexual desire and fantasies and improves mood in hypogonadal men. There appear to be important differences in the dose–response and sexual desire between younger and older men. Low-normal levels of testosterone appear to be enough to normalize the brain's erotic functions in younger men, but middle-aged and older men have dose-dependent increases in libido with higher dosages of testosterone. Contrary to popular belief, exogenous testosterone at dosages from normal physiological up to two to three times greater than physiological replacement does not induce aggressive behaviour. In fact, hypogonadal men report decreased tension, anger, and improved self-esteem after treatment with testosterone. Case reports of androgen-induced violence and anger are uncommon and almost always associated with abuse due to very high dosages of synthetic androgenic anabolic steroids.

13.3 **Effects in older men**

As men age, they have declining circulating testosterone levels and often have declining cognitive function, too. Because testosterone has been shown to have neuroprotective effects, it is tempting to speculate that testosterone may prevent cognitive decline and dementia. In older men with low-normal circulating testosterone levels, androgen supplementation at a high-normal replacement dosage causes significant improvements in tests of spatial and verbal memory. It has not been demonstrated that these cognitive improvements on experimental tests translate into clinically meaningful improvements. Similar to studies of younger hypogonadal men, the positive effects of high-normal replacement dosages of androgen on spatial memory appear to be mediated directly via an androgen effect, but the improvement in verbal memory is due to aromatization of androgen to oestrogen. Low dosages of testosterone supplementation may have little or no effect on cognition in older men with low-normal serum testosterone levels.

The effects of testosterone on cognition in older men may be affected by apolipoprotein E ε4 status. Apolipoprotein E ε4 is considered to be a major risk factor for Alzheimer's disease. In older men that are not apolipoprotein E ε4 carriers, higher serum testosterone levels are associated with better cognitive function, but higher circulating testosterone levels are associated with lower cognitive function in older men that are apolipoprotein E ε4 carriers.

13.3.1 **Androgen therapy and dementia**

In experimental studies, short-term testosterone administration has been shown to induce significant improvements in cognitive tests in older men with baseline low-normal testosterone levels and mild cognitive impairment due to Alzheimer's disease. There are no long-term studies of androgen therapy in older men with low or low-normal testosterone levels plus Alzheimer's disease, but it is unlikely that androgen supplementation will reverse moderate or severe dementia. Nonetheless, it is possible that androgen therapy may be useful in improving cognitive function and ability to perform activities of daily living in men with mild dementia.

13.3.2 **Prevention of dementia**

Although it is unlikely that testosterone therapy will play a significant part in the treatment of Alzheimer's disease in older men, it is possible that testosterone supplementation in older men with low or low-normal testosterone levels could prevent or delay the onset of Alzheimer's disease or other causes of dementia. The biological plausibility for this hypothesis includes the following androgenic effects: anti-glucocorticoid effects on neurons, neurotrophic effects, and inhibition of neuronal apoptosis. In addition, animal studies indicate that androgens may decrease the formation of amyloid β peptide, a major pathogenic factor in the development of Alzheimer's disease.

It must be noted that clinical trials examining the effects of post-menopausal hormone therapy on the prevention and treatment of Alzheimer's disease in women have been disappointing. We have too few data to determine whether androgen supplementation in older men will preserve or improve cognitive function.

13.4 Future directions for research

More studies need to be done on the cognitive effects of androgens and their metabolites in men. Specific, interesting, clinical syndromes for study include investigating (1) the effects of neonatal and early pubertal androgen therapy on brain development and intelligence in boys with Klinefelter's Syndrome, and (2) the effects of early treatment with androgen supplementation on the natural history of multiple sclerosis. In addition, there must be large clinical trials investigating whether androgen supplementation may prevent or delay Alzheimer's disease.

13.5 Recommendations

Testosterone should not be prescribed as primary therapy to treat major depression in men with low testosterone levels. It is reasonable to prescribe androgen therapy and assess clinical response before prescribing antidepressant therapy to mildly depressed hypogonadal men. In younger and older men who are clinically and biochemically hypogonadal, testosterone therapy consistently improves mood, vitality, and sexual desire.

Testosterone therapy should not be prescribed solely with the intent to treat or prevent dementia: however, testosterone has clinically important cognitive effects in hypogonadal men. Clinical observation suggests that hypogonadal men tend to concentrate better and have improved mental alertness after normalizing of circulating testosterone levels. The improvement in cognitive effects is greatest for men with very low baseline testosterone levels. There are conflicting data on the dosage effects of testosterone on cognition, but it appears that younger men have a relatively low 'ceiling effect' (no improvement in cognitive function at higher dosages of androgen therapy), whereas older men may benefit from high-normal androgen dosages.

13.6 **Conclusions**

Sex steroid hormones play an important part in brain development and in cognitive function throughout human male life. Androgen effects on the brain extend beyond the well known effects on sexual desire and include positive effects on visuospatial skills, working memory, and aspects of verbal memory. It is very unusual to induce aggressive or violent behaviour during the course of androgen therapy at typical androgen replacement dosages. Clinically, hypogonadal men often report improvement in mood, vigour, and mental acuity during androgen therapy. These positive effects on brain function are often the most significant benefits of androgen therapy in male hypogonadism.

Key references

Cherrier MM, Matsumoto AM, Amory JK, et al. (2005a). The role of aromatization in testosterone supplementation: effects on cognition in older men. *Neurology* **64**: 290–6.

Cherrier MM, Matsumoto AM, Amory JK, et al. (2005b). Testosterone improves spatial memory in men with Alzheimer disease and mild cognitive impairment. *Neurology* **64**: 2063–8.

Cherrier MM, Matsumoto AM, Amory JK, et al. (2007). Characterization of verbal and spatial memory changes from moderate to supraphysiological increases in serum testosterone in healthy older men. *Psychoneuroendocrinology* **32**: 72–9.

Emmelot-Vonk MH, Verhaar HJJ, Nakhai Pour HR, et al. (2008). Effect of testosterone supplementation on functional mobility, cognition, and other parameters in older men. *JAMA* **299**: 39–52.

Fuller SJ, Tan RS, Martins RN. (2007). Androgens in the etiology of Alzheimer's disease in aging men and possible therapeutic interventions. *J Alzheimers Dis* **12**: 129–42.

Martin DM, Wittert G, Burns NR, Haren MT, Sugarman R. (2007a). Testosterone and cognitive function in aging men: data from the Florey Adelaide Male Aging Study (FAMAS). *Maturitas* **57**: 182–94.

Martin DM, Wittert G, Burns NR. (2007b). Gonadal steroids and visuo-spatial abilities in adult males: implications for generalized age-related cognitive decline. *Aging Male* **10**: 17–29.

Zitzmann M. (2006). Testosterone and the brain. *Aging Male* **9**: 195–9.

Chapter 14

The role of androgens in osteoporosis and frailty

Karen Choong and Shalender Bhasin

Key points

- Ageing is associated with declines in skeletal muscle mass, muscle strength and power, physical function, and bone mass and quality; these impairments contribute to increased risk of falls, disability, and fractures.
- In epidemiological studies, low testosterone levels are associated with lower skeletal muscle mass, muscle strength, physical function, bone mineral density, and higher risk of functional limitations, fractures, and mortality.
- Testosterone therapy in older men with low and low-normal testosterone levels improves lean body mass and grip strength. However, the effects of testosterone on physical function and health-related outcomes in older men with functional limitations need further investigation.
- Testosterone promotes the differentiation of mesenchymal multipotent stem cells into the myogenic lineage by androgen receptor-mediated mechanisms.
- The long-term risks of testosterone administration on prostate and cardiovascular outcomes are unknown. Selective androgen receptor modulators that selectively increase muscle mass without affecting the prostate would be attractive as function-promoting therapies.

14.1 Ageing and its effects on muscle and bone

With increasing life expectancies in men and women, functional limitations and osteoporosis and their adverse consequences have been the focus of intense investigation. Ageing is associated with a selective, accelerated loss of fast-twitch, type II muscle fibres more than type I fibres, and an increased accumulation of connective tissue and intramuscular fat. Diminished strength, loss of power-generating capacity and muscle aerobic activity from loss of muscle mass all lead to compromised physical function. Sarcopenia, the age-related decline in muscle mass with associated loss of muscle strength, limits the ability of the elderly to participate in activities of daily living, contributes to impairments in gait and balance, and increases the risk of falls, fractures, and disability.

Bone mineral density also declines with advancing age and contributes to the increased risk of low trauma fractures in older individuals. Fractures in the hip and spine are associated with increased risk of subsequent morbidity, mortality, disability, and reduced quality of life. Ageing-related loss of muscle mass and strength also contribute to increased fall propensity and the risk of low trauma fracture. The substantial societal and economic consequences of osteoporosis in the elderly have been well documented.

Although age-related changes in musculoskeletal health are a consequence of a multitude of factors, including systemic inflammation, poor nutrition, decreased physical activity, and changes in the hormonal milieu, the changes in circulating testosterone levels are a remediable factor and the focus of this review.

14.2 **Age-related changes in the hypothalamic–pituitary–testicular axis**

Serum total and free testosterone levels decline in men with advancing age. As sex hormone binding globulin concentrations are higher in older men than in young men, the age-related decline in free and bioavailable testosterone concentrations is greater than the decline in total testosterone concentrations. The age-related decline in testosterone concentrations begins in the third decade of life, continues throughout life, and is affected by co-morbid conditions, medications, and adiposity. In the Baltimore Longitudinal Study of Aging (BLSA), 30% of men over the age of 60 and 50% of men over the age of 70 had total testosterone concentrations below the lower limit of the normal range for healthy young men (325 ng/dl, 11.3 nmol/l). The prevalence rates were even higher when these investigators used a free testosterone index to define androgen deficiency. Some reports suggest that circulating testosterone concentrations in men are in an age-independent, secular decline that cannot be explained by increasing body mass index and prevalence of obesity, other co-morbid conditions, or decreasing incidence of smoking.

The age-related decline in testosterone levels is the result of decreased testosterone production rates; the plasma clearance of testosterone is lower in older men than in young men. The decreased testosterone production rates in older men result from abnormalities at all levels of the hypothalamic–pituitary–testicular axis. Leydig cell mass is reduced and the testosterone response to luteinizing hormone (LH) is attenuated in older men. Serum LH and follicle-stimulating hormone concentrations are higher in older men than young men. However, the increase in serum LH concentrations is less than that expected from the age-related decline in circulating testosterone levels, probably due to the impairment of gonadotrophin-releasing hormone (GnRH) secretion and alterations in gonadal steroid feed-back and feed-forward relationships. Older men are more sensitive to the feedback inhibitory effects of testosterone on LH. Hypothalamic GnRH secretion is decreased in older men, pulsatile LH secretion becomes disorderly, and the synchrony between LH and testosterone secretion is attenuated. The prepro-GnRH mRNA content, the number of neurons expressing prepro-GnRH mRNA, and the GnRH content of several hypothalamic areas are lower in older male rats in comparison with young rats; this is presumably due to the decreased hypothalamic excitatory amino acid expression and the reduced responsiveness of GnRH neurons to N-methyl-D-aspartate.

In epidemiological studies of community dwelling older men, lower bioavailable testosterone concentrations are associated with lower lean body mass and strength of upper and lower extremity muscles. Low testosterone levels in older men are also associated with decreased self-reported physical function, lower performance scores in objective measures of physical function, and increased risk of falls. In the Longitudinal Aging Study of Amsterdam, serum testosterone concentrations were positively correlated with muscle strength and physical performance.

14.3 Low testosterone levels in chronic illness

The clinical course of many chronic illnesses (e.g. those associated with HIV infection, chronic obstructive lung disease, end-stage renal disease, congestive heart failure, untreated diabetes, and some types of cancers) is often complicated by loss of skeletal muscle mass, physical dysfunction, and a high prevalence of low testosterone levels. The loss of muscle mass in chronic illnesses is associated with an increased risk of functional limitations, loss of independence, impaired quality of life, and mortality.

High frequency of low testosterone levels has been found in all the chronic illnesses that have been investigated. Recent surveys have reported low testosterone levels in 20–30% of HIV-infected men on highly effective anti-retroviral drug therapy; 80% of HIV-infected men with low testosterone levels have low or low-normal LH levels and

20% have elevated LH levels, suggesting primary testicular dysfunction. Low testosterone levels in HIV-infected men are associated with low lean body mass, decreased exercise capacity, wasting, and more accelerated disease progression to AIDS. Fifty per cent of men with chronic obstructive lung disease and 50–70% of men with end-stage renal disease have testosterone levels in the hypogonadal range.

14.4 Intervention trials of testosterone effects on muscle mass, strength, and physical function

14.4.1 Trials in hypogonadal men

Androgen deficiency in men (both spontaneous and experimentally induced by administration of a GnRH agonist) is associated with decreased fat-free mass and higher fat mass. Meta-analysis of largely open-label trials reveals that testosterone therapy of healthy, hypogonadal men increases fat-free mass by an average 2.8 kg. Testosterone therapy also improves maximal voluntary strength, fractional muscle protein synthesis, and fatty acid oxidation in healthy hypogonadal men.

14.4.2 Testosterone trials in healthy, eugonadal men

Raising testosterone levels by the administration of supraphysiological doses of testosterone is associated with greater increments in fat-free mass, muscle size, and maximal voluntary strength than if placebo is used. The anabolic effects of testosterone are augmented by resistance exercise training and concomitant human growth hormone administration. The increments in fat-free mass, muscle size, and maximal voluntary strength in response to testosterone administration are highly correlated with testosterone dose and the circulating testosterone concentrations. Testosterone increases maximal voluntary strength and leg power, but does not affect fatigability or specific force. There is little evidence that androgens affect endurance measures, such as VO_{2max} or lactate threshold.

14.4.3 Testosterone trials in older men

Testosterone trials in community-dwelling, healthy older men with low or low-normal testosterone levels have reported consistent increases in fat-free mass and a decrease in fat mass. In a meta-analysis of randomized testosterone trials in middle-aged and older men, testosterone therapy was associated with a greater improvement in fat-free mass (+2.5 kg, 95% confidence interval 1.5 to 3.4 kg), grip strength (3.3 kg, 95% CI 0.7 to 5.8 kg) and self-reported physical function (0.5 SD, 95% CI, 0.3, 0.7 SDs) than placebo (Figure 14.1). Changes in muscle strength and performance-based measures of

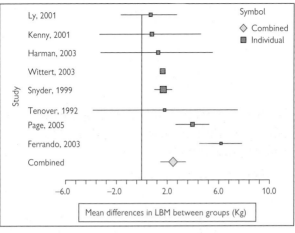

Figure 14.1a Forest plot of contrast in fat-free mass change between placebo and testosterone groups in randomized testosterone trials in healthy men 45 years of age and older. The systematic review included placebo-controlled randomized trials of testosterone administration for ≥90 days in healthy men 45 years of age or older men with low or low-normal testosterone levels that used testosterone or its esters in replacement doses, which also measured body composition. Odds ratios were pooled using a random effects model, assuming heterogeneous results across studies, after weighting for sample size. The Clopper–Pearson method was used to compute 95% confidence intervals. Reproduced with permission from: Bhasin *et al.* (2006) Drug insight: testosterone and selective androgen receptor modulators as anabolic therapies for chronic illness and aging. *Nat Clin Pract Endocrinol Metab* **2(3):** 146–59.

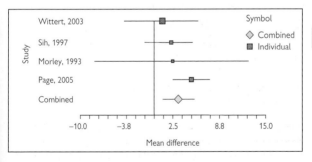

Figure 14.1b Forest plot of contrast in right-hand grip strength change between testosterone and placebo groups in randomized, placebo-controlled trials of testosterone administration in healthy men 45 years of age or older. Reproduced with permission from: Bhasin *et al.* (2006) Drug insight: testosterone and selective androgen receptor modulators as anabolic therapies for chronic illness and aging. *Nat Clin Pract Endocrinol Metab* **2(3):** 146–59.

physical function have been inconsistent across trials, although testosterone administration is associated with significant improvements in self-reported physical function, as assessed by the physical function domain of the SF-36 questionnaire.

The failure of the first-generation studies to demonstrate improvements in physical function in spite of a significant increase in fat-free mass is perplexing. These studies were relatively small and may have lacked adequate power to detect small but clinically important changes in physical function measures. The testosterone doses used in these studies were relatively small and were associated with relatively small gains in muscle mass; additionally, the men included in these earlier trials were not uniformly hypogonadal. The measures of physical function used in these studies suffered from a low ceiling effect; it is possible that the asymptomatic, healthy older men included in these studies had baseline muscle strength that was far higher than the threshold below which these measures would detect impairment. The effects of testosterone administration on health-related outcomes have not been investigated especially in older men with symptomatic functional limitations.

14.4.4 **Testosterone trials in HIV-infected men with weight loss**

A number of trials have examined the effects of androgen therapy in HIV-infected men with weight loss using a variety of androgens, including testosterone, nandrolone decanoate, oxandrolone, and oxymetholone. In one such study (meta-analysis of randomized, placebo-controlled trials of testosterone therapy of 3–6 months in HIV-infected men with weight loss) testosterone supplementation was associated with greater gains in lean body mass than with placebo administration (difference in lean body mass change between placebo and testosterone therapy 1.22 kg, 95% CI 0.23 to 2.22 for the random effect model) (Figure 14.2). In some trials that measured muscle strength, testosterone administration significantly improved maximal voluntary strength. Testosterone administration had a positive effect on depression indices (–0.6, 95% CI –1.0, –0.2). Testosterone effects on physical function, risk of disability, disease progression, and long-term safety in men with HIV infection need further investigation.

Testosterone therapy has generally been safe; the frequency of adverse events did not differ significantly between the testosterone and placebo groups. There were no significant changes in CD4+ T lymphocyte counts, HIV copy number, PSA, and plasma high-density lipoprotein cholesterol. Thus, 3–6 months of testosterone administration in HIV-infected men with low testosterone levels and weight loss can induce modest gains in body weight, lean body mass, and strength. Based on these data an Expert Panel of the Endocrine Society suggested

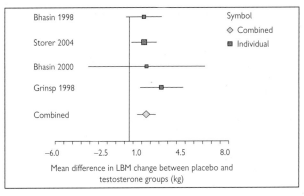

Figure 14.2 Forest plot of contrast in lean body mass between placebo and testosterone groups in randomized, placebo-controlled trials of testosterone administration in HIV-infected men with weight loss and low or low-normal testosterone levels. Reproduced with permission from: Bhasin *et al.* (2006) Drug insight: testosterone and selective androgen receptor modulators as anabolic therapies for chronic illness and aging. *Nat Clin Pract Endocrinol Metab* **2(3)**: 146–59.

that clinicians consider short-term testosterone therapy as an adjunctive therapy in HIV-infected men with low testosterone levels and weight loss to promote weight maintenance and gains in lean body mass (LBM) and muscle strength.

14.4.5 Testosterone supplementation in glucocorticoid-treated men

Skeletal muscle atrophy, osteoporosis, and the suppression of endogenous testosterone production are well known complications of glucocorticoid administration in pharmacological doses. In a meta-analysis of randomized, placebo-controlled trials, testosterone supplementation of men receiving glucocorticoid treatment for bronchial asthma or chronic obstructive pulmonary disease was associated with greater gain (contrast with placebo 2.3 kg, 95% CI 2.0, 3.6) in lean body mass and a greater decrease in fat mass (contrast −3.1 kg, 95% CI, −3.5, −2.8) than placebo. These trials showed an increase in bone mineral density in the lumbar spine (+4%, 95% CI 2 to 7), but the effect on femoral bone density was not significant. The small sample size, high loss-to-follow-up rates in one study, and heterogeneity of inclusion criteria weaken these inferences.

Glucocorticoids increase protein catabolism and reduce protein synthesis. Glucocorticoids upregulate myostatin expression and inhibit ribosomal protein translation by inhibiting mTOR signalling by reduced phosphorylation of the downstream targets S6K1 and 4E-BP1. Testosterone downregulates glucocorticoid receptors in the skeletal muscle cells and attenuates glucocorticoid signalling.

14.4.6 **Testosterone trials in men with chronic obstructive lung disease**

Muscle wasting and dysfunction are correctable causes of functional limitations and disability in patients with chronic obstructive pulmonary disease. In a randomized trial, testosterone therapy increased fat-free mass, muscle size, and muscle strength to a greater extent than placebo. Testosterone and resistance exercise training when administered together were associated with greater gains in fat-free mass and strength than either intervention alone. In another placebo-controlled randomized trial, nandrolone was compared with placebo; these authors reported modest increases in lean body mass and respiratory muscle strength.

14.4.7 **Testosterone trials in patients with end-stage renal disease**

Almost two-thirds of men with end-stage renal disease have low testosterone levels because of multiple pathophysiological factors that suppress all components of the hypothalamic–pituitary–testicular axis. The decrease in testosterone levels is a potentially correctable cause of muscle loss and dysfunction in patients with end-stage renal disease. Androgens have been used for over three decades for the treatment of anaemia in patients with end-stage renal disease. In a randomized trial, nandrolone administration was associated with significant improvements in lean body mass, walking speed, and stair climbing time; the improvements in lean body mass were greater than those in the placebo group. Adequately powered studies are needed to determine the effects of androgen therapy on physical function, quality of life, erythropoietin use, and other clinically relevant outcomes.

14.5 **Mechanisms of androgen action on the skeletal muscle**

Testosterone induces hypertrophy of both type I and type II muscle fibres in a dose-dependent manner, and increases the number of satellite cells. Testosterone enhances differentiation of mesenchymal, multipotent cells into the myogenic lineage and inhibits their differentiation into the adipocyte lineage through its binding to androgen receptor. Testosterone binding to androgen receptor promotes its association with its co-activator β-catenin, causing its translocation into the nucleus where it is associated with TCF-4 and activates a number of Wnt-target genes, including follistatin. Testosterone also stimulates muscle protein synthesis and reutilization of amino acids.

14.6 **Testosterone and osteoporosis**

Osteoporosis is a skeletal disorder characterized by decreased bone strength and increased risk of low trauma fracture, and is a major public health problem; 2 million American men have osteoporosis, and another 12 million are at risk for this disease. Although osteoporosis is less prevalent in men than in women, it is associated with substantial morbidity and greater excess mortality in men than in women. Osteoporosis in men remains underdiagnosed and suboptimally treated.

14.6.1 **Sex steroids and pubertal bone accretion**

Sex steroids play an important role in peri-pubertal bone accretion, epiphyseal fusion at the end of pubertal growth, and in the maintenance of bone mass throughout adult life. Androgen deficiency that develops before the completion of pubertal development is associated with reduced cortical and trabecular bone mass. During the pubertal years, significant bone accretion occurs under the influence of sex steroids; therefore, individuals with sex-steroid deficiency before or during peri-pubertal years may end up with suboptimal peak bone mass.

14.6.2 **Sex steroids and bone health in adult men**

Similarly, adult men with acquired androgen deficiency due to disorders of the hypothalamus, pituitary, or the testes have lower bone mineral density than age-matched controls. Men receiving androgen deprivation therapy for the treatment of prostate cancer experience accelerated bone loss and are at increased risk of low trauma fractures. Consistent with human data, androgen receptor knockout mice have lower bone mass than wild-type littermates.

14.6.3 **Age-related changes in sex hormones and bone health**

147

Age-related decline in sex hormones is associated with changes in bone mineral density, bone geometry, strength, and quality, and increased risk of osteoporotic fractures. Fifty per cent of older men with hip fractures have low testosterone levels as compared with 20% of age-matched controls without hip fracture. In epidemiological studies, bioavailable testosterone, total oestradiol, and bioavailable oestradiol levels are more strongly associated with bone mineral density of the spine, hip, and distal radius than total testosterone levels. In addition to the age-related changes in sex hormones, ageing is associated with loss of muscle mass and strength, which contribute to increased fall propensity.

14.6.4 **Effects of testosterone therapy on bone density and quality**

Testosterone replacement in healthy young hypogonadal men is associated with significant increases in vertebral bone mineral density. A meta-analysis of randomized trials revealed that testosterone replacement in relatively healthy older men increases vertebral bone mineral density; however, changes in femoral bone mineral density did not differ significantly between testosterone and placebo groups. Testosterone therapy in androgen-deficient men also improves trabecular architecture in addition to increasing bone mineral density. Adequately powered trials to determine the effects of testosterone therapy on fractures have not been conducted.

14.6.5 **Clinical implications**

Men who experience low trauma fracture, especially those below the age of 50, should be evaluated for androgen deficiency. The Endocrine Society Guidelines suggest that bone mineral density of the lumbar spine, femoral neck, and hip should be measured in all androgen-deficient men at baseline, and repeated after 1–2 years of testosterone therapy in hypogonadal men with osteoporosis or low trauma fracture. Selective oestrogen receptor modulators or bisphosphonates may be considered in men receiving androgen deprivation therapy for prostate cancer in whom androgen administration is contraindicated.

14.7 **Mechanisms by which testosterone regulates bone mass**

Short-term studies of androgen replacement have shown inconsistent increases in markers of bone formation, but a more consistent reduction in markers of bone resorption. Testosterone increases bone mineral density in part through its aromatization to oestrogen, which inhibits bone resorption. Thus, men with naturally occurring mutations of oestrogen receptor-α or CYP19 aromatase gene have delayed epiphyseal fusion and decreased bone mass. In men, androgens and oestrogens both play independent roles in regulating bone resorption. Oestrogens regulate the activation frequency of bone functional basic multicellular units, the duration of the resorption phase and the formation phase, and osteoclast recruitment. The protective effects of oestrogen on bone in both male and female mice during growth and maturation are mediated largely through oestrogen receptor-α. Testosterone might also directly stimulate osteoblastic bone formation. Androgen receptors have been demonstrated on osteoblasts and on mesenchymal stem cells. Testosterone stimulates cortical bone formation. Testosterone also stimulates the production of several growth factors, such as insulin-like growth factor 1, within the bone that may contribute to bone formation. Testosterone increases muscle mass and muscle strength, which may indirectly increase bone mass by increased loading. Testosterone might inhibit apoptosis of osteoblasts through non-genotropic mechanisms.

14.8 Selective androgen receptor modulators

Concerns about the long-term risks of prostate and cardiovascular disorders in older men treated with testosterone have encouraged efforts to develop selective androgen receptor modulators (SARM) that have the desired anabolic effects on the muscle, but that do not have adverse effects on prostate and cardiovascular outcomes. These non-steroidal SARMs do not serve as substrates for CYP19 aromatase or 5α-reductase, but act as full agonists in muscle and bone and as partial agonists in prostate and seminal vesicles. Structural modifications of aryl propionamide analogues, bicalutamide and hydroxyflutamide, led to the discovery of the first generation of SARMs. SARM pharmacophores can be classified into four categories: aryl-propionamide, bicyclic hydantoin, quinoline, and tetrahydroquinoline analogues.

The mechanisms of the tissue-selective actions of SARMs are poorly understood, although several have been proposed. Ligand binding induces specific conformational changes in the ligand-binding domain, which could modulate surface topology and subsequent protein–protein interactions between androgen receptors and other coregulators involved in genomic transcriptional activation or cytosolic proteins involved in non-genomic signalling. Differences in ligand-specific receptor conformation and protein–protein interactions could result in tissue-specific gene regulation, due to potential changes in interactions with the androgen response element (ARE), coregulators, or transcription factors.

First-generation SARMs act as full agonists in anabolic organs such as muscle and bone, while only as partial agonists in others, such as prostate tissue. In animal studies using castrated and aged-male rats, SARM administration improves bone mineral density and restores castration-induced loss in lean body mass, while having minimal effects on prostate growth. Hence, the preferential anabolic effects of SARMs on the muscle and bone hold considerable promise for their development as treatment options for osteoporosis and ageing-related functional limitations.

14.9 **Conclusions**

Ageing is associated with an increased risk of functional limitations, disability, falls, osteoporosis, and fractures. Testosterone increases skeletal muscle mass, maximal voluntary strength, and leg power, but does not affect fatigability or specific tension. Further studies are needed to determine whether testosterone therapy can improve physical function and health-related outcomes in older men with functional limitations. Testosterone administration increases vertebral bone mineral density, but the effects of testosterone therapy on fracture risk have not been studied. The long-term risks of testosterone therapy especially on prostate and cardiovascular outcomes are unknown.

Key references

Baumgartner RN, Koehler KM, Gallagher D, Romero L, Heymsfield SB, Ross RR, Garry PJ, Lindeman RD. (1998). Epidemiology of sarcopenia among the elderly in New Mexico. *Am J Epidemiol* **147**: 755–63.

Bhasin S, Storer TW, Berman N, Callegari C, Clevenger B, Phillips J, Bunnell TJ, Tricker R, Shirazi A, Casaburi R. (1996). The effects of supra-physiologic doses of testosterone on muscle size and strength in normal men. *N Engl J Med* **335**: 1–7.

Bhasin S, Woodhouse L, Casaburi R, Singh AB, Bhasin D, Berman N, Chen X, Yarasheski KE, Magliano L, Dzekov C, Dzekov J, Bross R, Phillips J, Sinha-Hikim I, Shen R, Storer TW. (2001). Testosterone dose-response relationships in healthy young men. *Am J Physiol Endocrinol Metab* **281**: E1172–81.

Bhasin S, Calof OM, Storer TW, Lee ML, Mazer NA, Jasuja R, Montori VM, Gao W, Dalton JT. (2006a). Drug Insight: testosterone and selective androgen receptor modulators as anabolic therapies for chronic illness and aging. *Nat Clin Pract Endocrinol Metab* **2**: 146–59.

Bhasin S, Cunningham GR, Hayes FJ, Matsumotot AM, Snyder PJ, Swerd-loff RS, Montori VM. (2006b). Testosterone therapy in adult men with androgen deficiency syndromes: an endocrine society clinical practice guideline. *J Clin Endocrinol Metab* **91**: 1995–2010.

Feldman HA, Longcope C, Derby CA, Johannes CB, Araujo AB, Coviello AD, Bremner WJ, McKinlay JB. (2002). Age trends in the level of serum testosterone and other hormones in middle-aged men: longitudinal results from the Massachusetts male aging study. *J Clin Endocrinol Metab* **87**: 589–98.

Harman SM, Metter EJ, Tobin JD, Pearson J, Blackman MR. (2001). Longitudinal effects of aging on serum total and free testosterone levels in healthy men. Baltimore Longitudinal Study of Aging. *J Clin Endocrinol Metab* **86**: 724–31.

Riggs BL, Khosla S, Melton LJ. (2002). Sex steroids and the construction and conservation of the adult skeleton. *Endocrine Rev* **23**: 279–302.

Chapter 15

A perspective from primary care

Douglas Savage and Trudy Hannington

Key points

- Hypogonadism, particularly late-onset hypogonadism is a common condition that is underdiagnosed.
- The primary care physician is ideally placed to make the initial diagnosis.
- It is important that the diagnosis and underlying cause is established by a specialist primary care physician or appropriate secondary care specialist.
- Testosterone replacement therapy can transform peoples lives, significantly improving quality of life of the individual and also their families.
- Therapy can also save marriages and partnerships.

15.1 Its not all about sex!

The following statement was written by a patient in the UK:

> The battle regarding the need to treat testosterone deficiency patients has raged for many years. It continues today, with an increasingly aware body of patients trying to obtain treatment from a seemingly unwilling medical community. Are these men pursuing 'boy-racer, sex machine' status in middle age? The answer is no. These are men who are trying to recover a semblance of normality. Libido tends to become a secondary issue when the balance of ones mind and body are disturbed.

How sadly true a statement is that. You will read a lot of the scientific argument about the reality and importance of late-onset hypogonadism. You are probably like I used to be in believing that hypogonadism was a rare condition and to be very much left to the secondary care endocrinologist. I hope to try and convince you that this is one of the most exciting areas of medicine today that can be diagnosed fairly easily in general practice. Please remember that having a low testosterone level is not good for your health, with several studies demonstrating that low testosterone status is associated with an increase in all-cause mortality by up to 68%. The diagnosis is not always straight forward, especially in men with borderline levels of testosterone, and there is also the potential for missing a very serious condition, such as a pituitary tumour; therefore most cases need to be referred to a specialist GP or secondary care for a definitive opinion.

15.2 Clinical awareness

My cynical teenage daughter once remarked 'seems to me you GPs don't do anything for anybody – you tell us patients that your symptoms are either due to your age or a virus'. How often that thought goes through my head on a bad day in general practice or as I am tending to find nowadays that much of the interesting work in general practice, adjustments of medication to help your patients with chronic disease lead healthy longer lives, is being managed in nurse-led special clinics for diabetes, cardiovascular disease, and asthma. So colleagues please become aware of patients who may well be suffering from hypogonadism and in particular late-onset hypogonadism – there are a lot of them out there especially those with metabolic syndrome, type 2 diabetes, significant truncal obesity, and those complaining of reduced libido or erectile dysfunction.

15.3 The size of the problem

Studies have found that 6–12% of men aged 40–70 years have low testosterone levels with associated clinical signs and symptoms. The HIM (hypogonadism in males) study estimated a prevalence of hypogonadism in men over 45 years in primary care practices. Of the 2162 men evaluated, 36.3% had low testosterone (<10.4 nmol/l). A further 80 were already receiving treatment for hypogonadism. Specific patient groups that have been found to have a high prevalence of low testosterone levels include those with type 2 diabetes, coronary heart disease, and osteoporotic fractures.

152

15.4 Symptoms that should alert the general practitioner to hypogonadism

Reduced or complete loss of libido is the major trigger to assess testosterone status; however, tiredness is a common complaint. So remember to check testosterone levels in men complaining of unexplained fatigue whose routine bloods have failed to find a cause, and to specifically ask about any sexual dysfunction as most men will not volunteer this information unless specifically asked.

The most common associated risk factors in a study of 520 men presenting with erectile dysfunction were hypertension (39%), hypogonadism (37%), and multiple medication (34%). Testosterone levels (as recommended by several national and international medical societies) should be assessed in all patients with erectile dysfunction.

In addition, many elderly men with depression are found to be hypogonadal.

15.5 **Testosterone replacement therapy**

Remember, before starting therapy all patients should have their testosterone levels checked on at least two separate occasions before 11.00 h. If the first test is abnormal then sex hormone binding globulin, follicle-stimulating hormone, luteinizing hormone, and prolactin should be measured with the second sample. It is important to look for an underlying cause. The patient should be counselled before commencing testosterone therapy and should have a rectal examination and prostate-specific antigen assayed before treatment to exclude any subclinical prostate cancer. Doctors in general in the past held the view that testosterone therapy increases the risk of developing prostate cancer. There is little evidence to support this and many studies have found that aggressive prostate cancers more often occur in patients with low testosterone levels.

The first choice therapy nowadays for many patients is testosterone gel with three preparations currently available for use in the UK. It is very important that men on testosterone therapy are kept under clinical observation. They should be reviewed every 3 months for the first year of treatment then yearly thereafter. At each visit full blood count and prostate-specific antigen should be measured.

15.6 **Awareness among clinicians**

For my ongoing education and to keep me up to date in the field of sexual medicine and andrology, I attend European conferences and read journals in this field. It is to my amazement and shock that most of our secondary care consultants in endocrinology and diabetology still don't seem to be fully aware of this condition or wish to accept it. Therefore, as a GP you can be in a very difficult situation of making an initial diagnosis, referring to secondary care, and finding to your surprise that patients with these typical symptoms and total testosterone levels between 8 and 10 nmol/l are told they have no hormonal abnormality. I have actually seen patients in our clinic with such a story and the patient is so relieved and thrilled when they are treated. Their symptoms improve because of course the worst thing was they felt as if they were neurotic and imagining their symptoms.

Finally, I would like to ask the Leger Clinic's Psychosexual Therapist Trudy Hannington to give a story of a couple that was referred to her.

15.7 **Case report**

Dave and Jenny were referred by his general practitioner to The Leger Clinic for psychosexual therapy in December 2006. Dave had lost his desire for sex.

This had been an ongoing problem for over 2 years and was now having a huge negative impact on his relationship with his wife. Dave was 47 years old, worked full-time and had two children. By the time Dave had sought help by going to see his doctor the marriage had almost broken down completely.

Previous blood tests performed by the general practitioner had all been reported as normal. The couple had had a number of sessions with marriage counsellors without any success.

During the initial consultation Dave admitted to being able to get an erection but was unable to maintain it. He also stated that even when he did get an erection he never had any desire to do anything with it! He never masturbated and could only have sex if he 'psyched himself up.' This would only happen on his wife's birthday and their wedding anniversary. After further discussion, Dave stated that on reflection his desire had always been low but in the last 2 years it had become non-existent.

His wife was extremely distressed and felt rejected. She had on some occasions blamed herself, believing that her husband no longer found her attractive, despite his attempts at reassurance. They no longer slept in the same bed and all basic intimacy had stopped. They both commented that they argued most of the time and Jenny had gone as far as seeing a solicitor and was considering a divorce.

On further questioning Dave revealed that he felt that he lacked in upper body strength, and that he could fall asleep if he just sat down for a minute. His wife commented that he had become 'old before his time.' There had been occasions when his wife thought that maybe he was being sexual with someone else even though there was no evidence to support this. However, Dave stated that he didn't even look at anyone else or ever felt attracted to anyone else. They both commented that the atmosphere in the house was strained and that they only did things as a family. They no longer went out as a couple and at all costs avoided planning nights out, or weekends away where they would be alone.

At the end of the assessment it was agreed that blood tests would be carried out, in particular to look at his testosterone levels. Once again the blood results were reported as 'normal' with a testosterone result of 9.0 nmol/l.

In the first session Dave and Jenny were given some suggestions that might enable them to start the process of introducing some basic intimacy, e.g. planning time together, kisses and cuddles, sitting on the same sofa, holding hands, etc. However, despite Dave complying with the suggestions he openly admitted that while it was quite pleasant to feel a little closer and have the pressure of sex lifted, he hadn't felt any enthusiasm or motivation to do more.

The second testosterone result was 9.8 nmol/l at the lower end of normal (normal range 8.4–30). A therapeutic trial of testosterone replacement therapy was commenced after agreement with Dave. Dave and Jenny returned to the clinic a week after starting treatment and Dave reported that he was experiencing morning erections, he felt he had more energy and that the world seemed to now be presenting itself in colour rather than 'black and white.' However, despite feeling sexual he had not acted on it. They both commented that because it had been so long they were both extremely anxious and nervous to start anything. Jenny stated that she also still felt a lot of resentment towards her husband for the constant rejection she had experienced.

A further hurdle that they needed to overcome was Dave returning to the marital bed.

Dave and Jenny attended for six psychosexual therapy sessions over a 3-month period, where issues of resentment were addressed, a sexual growth programme was introduced, basic intimacy established, and further encouragement to plan and prepare for intimate time together.

By the last session they were having regular sex and Dave admitted to thinking about sex much more. They no longer felt nervous about being alone together or planning nights and weekends away! They commented that 'we had saved their marriage' and were 'staggered by the improvements all round.' Dave commented that he actually felt sad that he had missed out on so much, never realizing what 'normal' felt like.

One of the biggest impacts was on the family as a whole. Their two children had commented directly to their parents that seeing mum and dad getting on had made them feel much happier and secure and that the atmosphere in the home was so much better. Dave and Jenny commented that what the children were now having difficulties with was seeing their parents 'so loved up!'

15.8 Conclusions

So you see you can make such a difference to patients' lives. Please be on the lookout for patients with late-onset hypogonadism, and, remember your diagnosis may well be correct with total testosterone levels between 8 and 12 nmol/l, given as within the 'normal range'.

Key references

Lazarou S, Morgentaler A. (2005). Hypogonadism in the man with erectile dysfunction: what to look for and when to treat. *Curr Urol Rep* **6**: 476–81.

Mulligan T, Frick MF, Zuraw QC, Stemhagen A, McWhirter C. (2006). Prevalence of hypogonadism in males aged at least 45 years: the HIM study. *Int J Clin Pract* **60**: 762–9.

Index

157